Pre Test®

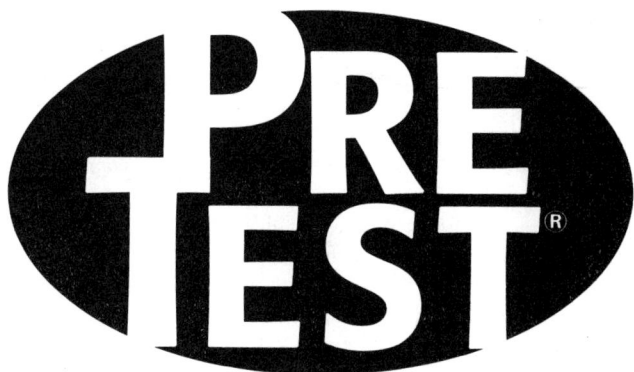

Clinical Vignettes
for the USMLE Step 1

PreTest® Self-Assessment and Review

NOTICE

Medicine is an ever-changing science. As new research and clinical experience broaden our knowledge, changes in treatment and drug therapy are required. The editors and the publisher of this work have checked with sources believed to be reliable in their efforts to provide information that is complete and generally in accord with the standards accepted at the time of publication. However, in view of the possibility of human error or changes in medical sciences, neither the editors nor the publisher nor any other party who has been involved in the preparation or publication of this work warrants that the information contained herein is in every respect accurate or complete, and they are not responsible for any errors or omissions or for the results obtained from use of such information. Readers are encouraged to confirm the information contained herein with other sources. For example and in particular, readers are advised to check the product information sheet included in the package of each drug they plan to administer to be certain that the information contained in this book is accurate and that changes have not been made in the recommended dose or in the contraindications for administration. This recommendation is of particular importance in connection with new or infrequently used drugs.

PRE TEST ®

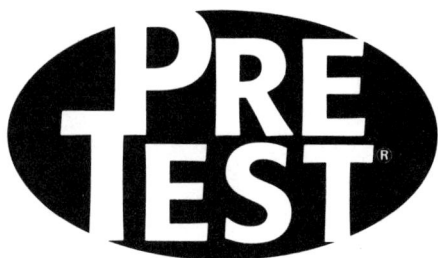

Clinical Vignettes
for the USMLE Step 1
PreTest® Self-Assessment and Review

McGraw-Hill
Health Professions Division
PreTest® Series

NEW YORK   ST. LOUIS   SAN FRANCISCO   AUCKLAND
BOGOTÁ   CARACAS   LISBON   LONDON   MADRID
MEXICO CITY   MILAN   MONTREAL   NEW DELHI
SAN JUAN   SINGAPORE   SYDNEY   TOKYO   TORONTO

McGraw-Hill

A Division of The **McGraw·Hill** *Companies*

Clinical Vignettes for the USMLE Step I: PreTest® Self-Assessment and Review

1 2 3 4 5 6 7 8 9 0   DOCDOC   9 9

ISBN 0-07-135133-7

This book was set in Berkeley by V & M Graphics.
The editors were John J. Dolan and Peter McCurdy.
Project development was by Joanna V. Pomeranz, V & M Graphics.
The production supervisor was Helene G. Landers.
The text designer was Jim Sullivan/RepoCat Graphics & Editorial Services.
The cover designer was Li Chen Chang / Pinpoint.
R.R. Donnelley & Sons was printer and binder.

This book is printed on acid-free paper.

CONTENTS

PREFACE

The current format of the United States Medical Licensing Exam for Step 1 emphasizes clinical vignettes as the primary test question. The exam is 350 questions, broken up into 7 blocks of 50 questions each. Students have approximately one hour to finish each exam.

Clinical Vignettes for the USMLE Step 1 parallels this format. The book is 350 questions of clinical vignettes covering all of the basic sciences. The questions are divided into 7 blocks of 50 questions. Halfway through each block, a stopwatch set at 30 minutes is included to remind the student of the one hour limit for each block. Answers are comprehensive and referenced to major texts and journals, a trademark of the PreTest® series. Because this book so closely follows the Step 1 exam, we recommend that students finish one block in an hour, rest, and then proceed to the next block as if they were actually sitting for the exam.

These questions were taken from the 11 PreTest® Basic Science books and were edited as needed to reflect the current USMLE format. The Publisher acknowledges and thanks the following authors for their contributions to this book:

Ernest W. April, Anatomy
Evan G. Pattishal, Jr., Behavioral Sciences
Francis J. Chlapowski, Biochemistry
Golder M. Wilson, Genetics
Robert M. Klein and James C. McKenzie, Histology and Cell Biology
Richard C. Tilton, Microbiology
Allan Siegel and Heidi Siegel, Neuroscience
Earl Brown, Pathology
Maurice A. Mufson, Pathophysiology
Arnold Stern, Pharmacology
James P. Ryan and Ronald F. Tuma, Physiology
In addition, the publisher thanks Joanna V. Pomeranz, V & M Graphics, for her development work on this project.

McGraw-Hill
March, 1999

BLOCK I

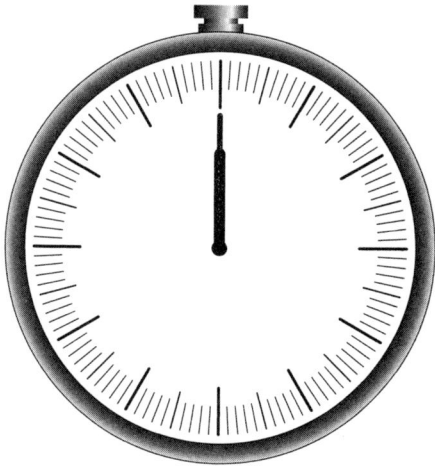

YOU HAVE **60** MINUTES
TO COMPLETE **50** QUESTIONS.

BLOCK I

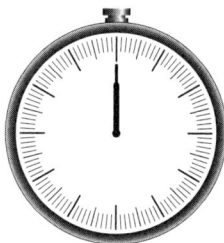

YOU HAVE *60* MINUTES
TO COMPLETE *50* QUESTIONS.

Questions

1-1. A 4-year-old female is being evaluated for the sudden onset of multiple petechiae and bruises. She is found to have a peripheral leukocyte count of 55,000, 86 percent of which are small, homogeneous cells that have nuclei with immature chromatin. Indistinct nucleoli are also present. Initial tests on these immature cells are as follows: TdT positive, PAS positive, acid phosphatase positive, and myeloperoxidase negative. Based on these findings, the immature cells most likely originated from

a. Myeloblasts
b. Monoblasts
c. Megakaryoblasts
d. Lymphoblasts
e. Erythroblasts

1-2. A 6-year-old boy has received a deep puncture wound while playing in his neighbor's yard. His records indicate that he has had the standard DPT (diphtheria, pertussis, tetanus) immunizations and a booster when he entered school. What is the most appropriate therapy for this child?

a. Tetanus toxoid
b. Tetanus antitoxin
c. Both toxoid and antitoxin at the same site
d. Toxoid and antitoxin at different sites
e. No treatment

Clinical Case (Questions 1-3 through 1-6)

Helen is a 76-year-old woman who has had high blood pressure and dia-betes for more than ten years. One day, as she was reaching for a jar of flour in order to make an apple pie, her right side suddenly gave out and she collapsed. While trying to get up from the floor, she noticed that she was unable to move her right arm or leg. Helen attempted to cry for help because she was unable to reach the telephone; however, her speech was slurred and rather unintelligible. She lay on the floor and waited for help to arrive.

Helen's son began to worry about his usually prompt mother when she didn't arrive with her apple pie. After several attempts at telephoning her apartment without an answer, he drove to her apartment and found her lying on the floor. She attempted to tell him what had happened, but her speech was too slurred to comprehend, so assuming his mother had had a stroke, her son called an ambulance to bring her to the nearest emer-gency room.

A neurology resident was called to see Helen in the emergency room because the physicians there, too, felt she had had a stroke. The resident noted that Helen followed commands very well, and although her speech was very slurred, it was fluent and grammatically correct. The lower two thirds of her face drooped on the right, but when asked to raise her eye-brows, her forehead appeared symmetric. Her tongue pointed to the right side when she was asked to protrude it. Her right arm and leg were severe-ly but equally weak, but her left side had normal strength. She felt a pin and a vibrating tuning fork equally on both sides.

1-3. Where in the central nervous system did Helen's stroke occur?

a. Left precentral gyrus
b. Right precentral gyrus
c. Left basilar pons or left internal capsule
d. Right putamen or globus pallidus
e. Left thalamus

1-4. A computed tomography (CT) scan revealed a new infarct in the left internal capsule. Which artery was occluded, causing the stroke?

a. Lenticulostriate branches of the middle cerebral artery
b. Posterior cerebral artery
c. Anterior cerebral artery
d. Vertebral artery
e. Posterior choroidal artery

I-5. Damage to which two tracts caused Helen to be weak on her right side?

a. Spinothalamic and corticospinal tracts
b. Spinothalamic and corticobulbar tracts
c. Corticospinal and corticobulbar tracts
d. Corticospinal and spinocerebellar tracts
e. Corticospinal and rubrospinal tracts

I-6. Helen's forehead is spared from the weakness because

a. The forehead is innervated by different fibers originating in the postcentral gyrus.
b. There are two cranial nerves innervating the forehead.
c. The forehead is represented bilaterally at the cortical level.
d. The forehead is stronger than the rest of the face.
e. Thalamic regions receiving inputs from the forehead contain few inhibitory neurons.

I-7. A 14-month-old male infant presents with an enlarging abdominal mass. Laboratory examination reveals increased urinary levels of metanephrine and VMA (vanillylmandelic acid). A histologic section from this mass reveals a tumor composed of small primitive-appearing cells with hyperchromatic nuclei and little to no cytoplasm. Occasional focal groups of tumor cells are arranged in a ring around a central space. What is the correct diagnosis for this tumor?

a. Adrenal cortical carcinoma
b. Ganglioneuroma
c. Nephroblastoma
d. Neuroblastoma
e. Pheochromocytoma

I-8. An 86-year-old male complains of cough and blood in his sputum for the past two days. On admission, his temperature is 103°F. Physical examination reveals rales in his right lung, and x-ray examination shows increased density in the right middle lobe. A sputum smear shows many Gram-positive cocci, confirmed by sputum culture as penicillinase-producing *Staphylococcus aureus*. Which of the following agents should be given?

a. Ampicillin
b. Oxacillin
c. Carbenicillin
d. Ticarcillin
e. Mezlocillin

1-9. A 49-year-old female patient is being treated with penicillin for acute salpingitis and pelvic inflammatory disease without benefit. Which of the following organisms should now be considered in the differential diagnosis?

a. *Treponema pallidum*
b. *Neisseria gonorrhoeae*
c. *Chlamydia trachomatis*
d. Adenoviruses
e. Herpesviruses

1-10. A 37-year-old woman complained of prolonged cramps, nausea, vomiting, diarrhea, and episodic flushing of the skin. At autopsy, pearly-white, plaque-like deposits were found on the tricuspid valve leaflets. These cardiac lesions most likely were due to

a. Rheumatic heart disease
b. Amyloidosis
c. Iron overload
d. Hypothyroidism
e. Carcinoid heart disease

1-11. A young couple, both in their 20s, have been trying for 2 years to have a baby. The man comes into the office and, on workup, has oligospermia, a high LH level, a high FSH level, and a normal karyotype. How do you treat him?

a. Do nothing.
b. Administer testosterone injections.
c. Check the partner for causes of infertility.
d. Counsel regarding infertility.

1-12. A 35-year-old male living in a southern region of Africa presents with increasing abdominal pain and jaundice. He has worked as a farmer for many years, and sometimes his grain has become moldy. Physical examination reveals a large mass involving the right side of his liver, and a biopsy specimen from this mass confirms the diagnosis of liver cancer (hepatocellular carcinoma). The pathogenesis of this tumor involves which of the following substances?

a. Aflatoxin B_1
b. Direct acting alkylating agents
c. Vinyl chloride
d. Azo dyes
e. Beta-naphthylamine

1-13. A married second year medical student with two young children is notified by her children's day care center that two other children at the day care center have recently been diagnosed as having viral hepatitis. Without any other information, this second year student correctly assumes that the most likely causative agent for these two cases of hepatitis is

a. Hepatitis A virus
b. Hepatitis B virus
c. Hepatitis C virus
d. Hepatitis D virus
e. Cytomegalovirus (CMV)

1-14. A 22-year-old male migrant farm worker in the San Joaquin Valley of California has been hospitalized for 2 weeks with progressive lassitude, fever of unknown origin, and skin nodules on the lower extremities. A biopsy of one of the deep dermal nodules shown in the photomicrograph below reveals the presence of

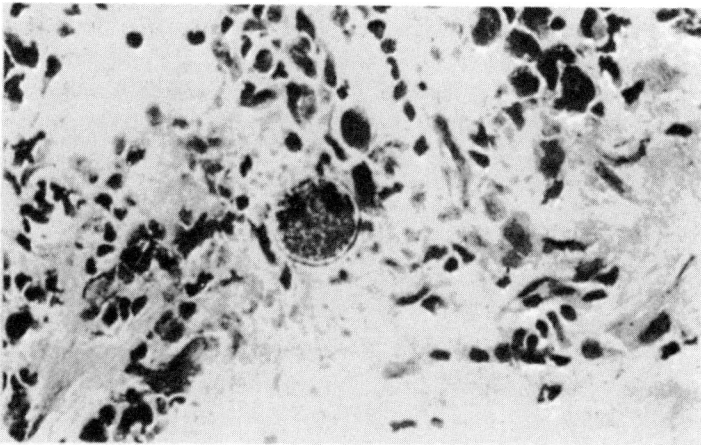

a. Russell bodies
b. Malignant lymphoma
c. Coccidioides spherule

d. Lymphomatoid granulomatosis
e. Erythema nodosum

1-15. A 25-year-old woman has amenorrhea and galactorrhea. The results of her thyroid function tests are normal. Her prolactin level is 350 µg/L (n <20). The most likely cause for her hyperprolactinemia is

a. Microadenoma
b. Macroadenoma
c. Antidepressant use
d. Exercise induced
e. Antihypertensive therapy

1-16. A 25-year-old woman with known systemic lupus erythematosus presents with jaundice, splenomegaly, peripheral blood schistocytes, and a reticulocyte count of 24 percent. The antibody most likely to be responsible for this complex reacts in vitro at

a. 5°C
b. 20°C
c. 25°C
d. 37°C
e. 56°C

1-17. A 55-year-old female presents with pain in her right hip and thigh. The pain started approximately 6 months ago and is a deep ache that worsens when she stands or walks. Your examination reveals increased warmth over the right thigh. The only laboratory abnormalities are alkaline phosphatase 656 IU/L (normal 23 to 110 IU/L), elevated 24-h urine hydroxyproline, and osteocalcin 13 ng/mL (normal <6 ng/mL). X-ray of hips and pelvis shows osteolytic lesions and regions with excessive osteoblastic activity. Bone scan shows significant uptake in the right proximal femur.

Which of the following would you include in your differential diagnosis?

a. Paget's disease
b. Multiple myeloma
c. Osteomalacia
d. Osteoporosis
e. Hypoparathyroidism

1-18. During an office visit, a 40-year-old female reports that she is awakened in the middle of the night by intense jaw pain and often is gritting or grinding her teeth. Relaxing the jaw does not help ease the pain. She is a very active, social, and energetic person. From your experience with previous patients suffering from temporomandibular disorders, you suspect that the primary causal link is

a. Muscular fatigue
b. Physical trauma
c. Muscular or joint infection
d. Anxiety or depression
e. Early rheumatoid arthritis

1-19. A 42-year-old female during a routine physical examination is found to have an elevated blood pressure of 150/100 mmHg. Work-up reveals a small left kidney and a normal-sized right kidney. Laboratory examination reveals elevated serum renin levels. Further work-up reveals that renal vein renin levels are increased on the left, but decreased on the right. This patient's hypertension is most likely the result of

a. Atherosclerotic narrowing of the left renal artery
b. Atherosclerotic narrowing of the right renal artery
c. Fibromuscular hyperplasia of the left renal artery
d. Fibromuscular hyperplasia of the right renal artery
e. Hyaline arteriolosclerosis

1-20. A 3-year-old child presents at the physician's office with symptoms of coryza, conjunctivitis, low-grade fever, and Koplik's spots. The causa-tive agent of this disease belongs to which group of viruses?

a. Adenovirus
b. Herpesvirus
c. Picornavirus
d. Orthomyxovirus
e. Paramyxovirus

1-21. A 25-year-old woman presents with increasing obesity, amenorrhea, hypertension, and abdominal stria. The next best diagnostic test is

a. Prolactin
b. Free T_4 and TSH
c. Overnight dexamethasone suppression
d. Random cortisol
e. Adrenocorticotropic hormone (ACTH)

Clinical Case (Questions 1-22 through 1-25)

Norma is a 75-year-old woman who had a stroke several months ago, manifested by numbness on her right side, including her arm, face, trunk, and leg. The numbness had improved somewhat over time, but did not completely disappear. One day, she noticed that brushing her right arm against a door was very painful. Thinking that perhaps this was "in her mind," she tried touching the right arm with her left hand, and this, too, was painful. Fearful that she may be having another stroke, she went immediately to see her neurologist at her local hospital.

Norma's neurologist examined her and found that sensation for a pin, temperature, and vibration were diminished on the entire right side of her body. The degree of sensory loss was unchanged from an examination several months before. However, she had a large amount of discomfort with any type of stimulus, accompanied by some emotional disturbance. The discomfort was far out of proportion to the degree of the stimulus; for instance, a light touch to her right arm would engender a scream similar to that elicited by a knife. The remainder of her examination was normal.

The neurologist told Norma that he didn't think that she had had a new stroke, but would order a head CT to be sure that there was no tumor or bleeding. In addition, he told her that if the head CT showed nothing new, that she could begin a new medication which would help with the pain.

1-22. What is the most likely location of the old stroke?

a. Right precentral gyrus
b. Left precentral gyrus
c. Right ventral thalamus
d. Left ventral thalamus
e. Left cerebral peduncle

1-23. Which two nuclei mediating sensation of the arms, face, legs, and trunk may have sustained damage from the original stroke?

a. Lateral and medial geniculate nuclei of the thalamus
b. Ventral posterior lateral and ventral posterior medial nuclei of the thalamus
c. Putamen and globus pallidus
d. Caudate and putamen
e. Anterior and lateral dorsal nuclei of the thalamus

1-24. Which pathway mediating pain is the afferent input into the infarcted area?

a. Tractus gracilis
b. Tractus cuneatus
c. Spinocerebellar tract
d. Spinothalamic tract
e. Corticospinal tract

1-25. Surgical stimulation of various regions of the central nervous system has been shown to alleviate pain. What is the location of one of these areas producing analgesia?

a. Anterior nucleus of the thalamus
b. Caudate nucleus
c. Anterior horn of the spinal cord
d. Globus pallidus
e. Periaqueductal gray

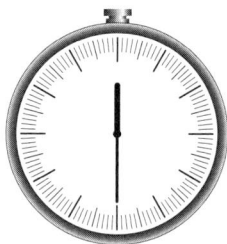

YOU SHOULD HAVE COMPLETED APPROXIMATELY
25 QUESTIONS AND HAVE 30 MINUTES REMAINING.

1-26. A 54-year-old male develops a thrombus in his left anterior descending coronary artery. The area of myocardium supplied by this vessel is irreversibly injured. The thrombus is destroyed by the infusion of streptokinase, which is a plasminogen activator, and the injured area is reperfused. The patient, however, develops an arrhythmia and dies. An electron microscopic (EM) picture taken from the irreversibly injured myocardium reveals the presence of large, dark, irregular amorphic densities. These flocculent densities are typically found within the

a. Golgi apparatus
b. Mitochondria
c. Nucleus
d. Rough endoplasmic reticulum
e. Smooth endoplasmic reticulum

1-27. A couple is referred to the physician because the first three pregnancies have ended in spontaneous abortion. Chromosomal analysis reveals that the wife has two cell lines in her blood, one with a missing X chromosome (45,X) and the other normal (46,XX). Her chromosomal constitution can be described as

a. Chimeric
b. Monoploid
c. Trisomic
d. Mosaic
e. Euploid

1-28. While moving furniture, an 18-year-old man experiences excruciating pain in his right groin. A few hours later he also develops pain in the umbilical region with accompanying nausea. At this point he seeks medical attention. Examination reveals a bulge midway between the midline and the anterior superior iliac spine, but superior to the inguinal ligament. On coughing or straining, the bulge increases and the inguinal pain intensifies. The bulge courses medially and inferiorly into the upper portion of the scrotum and cannot be reduced with the finger pressure of the examiner. It is decided that a medical emergency exists, and the patient is scheduled for immediate surgery.

Nausea and diffuse pain referred to the umbilical region in this patient most probably are due to

a. Compression of the genitofemoral nerve
b. Compression of the ilioinguinal nerve
c. Dilation of the inguinal canal
d. Incarceration of a loop of small bowel
e. Ischemic necrosis of the cremaster muscle

1-29. A 26-year-old female patient displays an ipsilateral paralysis of lateral gaze coupled with a contralateral hemiplegia. A lesion is most likely situated in the

a. Ventromedial medulla
b. Dorsomedial medulla
c. Ventrocaudal pons
d. Dorsorostral pons
e. Ventromedial midbrain

1-30. A 19-year-old male being treated for leukemia develops fever. You give agents that will cover bacterial, viral, and fungal infections. Two days later, he develops acute renal failure. Which drug was most likely responsible?

a. vancomycin
b. ceftazidime
c. amphotericin B
d. acyclovir

1-31. A 17-year-old male presents with a lesion on his face that measures approximately 1.5 cm in greatest dimension. He has a history of numerous similar skin lesions that have occurred mainly in sun-exposed areas. This present lesion is biopsied and reveals an invasive squamous cell carcinoma. This patient most probably has one type of a group of inherited diseases associated with unstable DNA and increased incidence of carcinoma. What is the diagnosis for this patient?

a. Xeroderma pigmentosa
b. Wiskott-Aldrich syndrome
c. Familial polyposis
d. Sturge-Weber syndrome
e. Multiple endocrine neoplasia, type I (MEN I)

1-32. A 4-year-old girl presents in the clinic with megaloblastic anemia and failure to thrive. Blood chemistries reveal orotic aciduria. Enzyme measurements of white blood cells reveal a deficiency of the pyrimidine biosynthesis enzyme orotate phosphoribosyltransferase and abnormally high activity of the enzyme aspartate transcarbamoylase. Which one of the following treatments will reverse all symptoms if carried out chronically?

a. Blood transfusion
b. White blood cell transfusion
c. Dietary supplements of phosphoribosyl pyrophosphate (PRPP)
d. Oral thymidine
e. Oral uridine

1-33. A 30-year-old man has pain in the left scrotum. What is currently valid concerning types of tumor?

a. Alpha fetoprotein (AFP) is only elevated in seminomas.
b. The half-life of AFP is 24 to 36 h.
c. Lactate dehydrogenase (LDH) is an important marker to follow tumor progression or regression.
d. Human chorionic gonadotropin-β subunit (β-hCG) is only elevated in seminoma.

1-34. A 56-year-old male presents with the sudden onset of excruciating pain. He describes the pain as beginning in the anterior chest, radiating to the back, and then moving downward into the abdomen. His blood pressure is found to be 160/115. Your differential diagnosis includes myocardial infarction; however, no changes are seen on his EKG, and you consider this to be less of a possibility. You obtain an X-ray of this patient's abdomen and discover a "double barrel" aorta. This abnormality is most likely a result of

a. A microbial infection
b. Loss of elastic tissue in the media
c. A congenital defect in the wall of the aorta
d. atherosclerosis of abdominal aorta
e. Abnormal collagen synthesis

1-35. A 24-year-old man who is being evaluated for infertility complains of recurrent sinusitis and a productive cough. He is found to be sterile, and situs inversus of his organs is noted. The most likely diagnosis for his pulmonary disease is

a. Asthma
b. Bronchiolitis
c. Bronchiectasis
d. Chronic bronchitis
e. Emphysema

1-36. A 45-year-old male takes simvastatin for hypercholesterolemia; however, his cholesterol level remains above target at maximal doses. Cholestyramine is added to the therapeutic regimen. What drug-drug interaction can occur?

a. The combination will not lower cholesterol more than either agent alone.
b. The combination causes elevated very-low-density lipoprotein (VLDL).
c. Cholestyramine inhibits gastrointestinal (GI) absorption of simvastatin.
d. Simvastatin is a direct antagonist of cholestyramine.

1-37. A 26-year-old man contracted viral influenza with an unremitting fever of 39.5°C (103°F) for 3 days. Since spermatogenesis cannot occur above a scrotal temperature of 35.5°C (96°F), he was left with no viable sperm on his recovery. The time required for spermatogenesis, spermiogenesis, and passage of viable sperm to the epididymis is approximately

a. 3 days
b 1 week
c. 5 weeks
d. 2 months
e. 4 months

1-38. A 45-year-old man presents because of frontal bossing and an enlarged nose, tongue, and jaw. He has doughy palms and spadelike fingers. The best screening test to establish the diagnosis is

a. random growth hormone
b. insulin-like growth factor (IGF-1)
c. TSH
d. prolactin
e. fasting blood sugar

Clinical Case (Questions 1-39 through 1-42)
Morris is a 79-year-old man who was brought to the emergency room (ER) because his family was worried that he suddenly was not using his right arm and leg, and seemed to have a simultaneous behavior change. He was unable to write a reminder note to himself, even with his left hand, and he put his shoes on the wrong feet. A neurologist was called to the ER to examine the patient. A loud bruit (pronounced *bru-e*; a rumbling sound) was heard with a stethoscope over the left carotid artery in his neck. When asked to show the neurologist his left hand, he pointed to his right hand, since it could not move. The neurologist asked him to add numbers, and he was unable to do this, despite having spent his life as a bookkeeper. Morris was unable to name the fingers on either hand, and he could not form any semblance of a letter, using his left hand. His eyes did not blink when the neurologist waved his hands close to Morris's eyes in the left temporal and right nasal visual fields. The right lower two thirds of his face drooped. There was some asymmetry of his reflexes between the right and left sides, and there was a positive Babinski response of his right toe.

1-39. Where in the central nervous system is the damage?

a. Right frontal and parietal lobes
b. Left frontal and parietal lobes
c. Right frontal lobe
d. Left frontal lobe
e. Right temporal lobe

1-40. Assuming that Morris had a stroke, which artery has become occluded?

a. Left anterior cerebral
b. Right anterior cerebral
c. Right middle cerebral
d. Left middle cerebral
e. Left posterior cerebral

1-41. Damage to which area of the brain caused Morris's inability to move his right side?

a. Right precentral gyrus
b. Left precentral gyrus
c. Right angular gyrus
d. Left angular gyrus
e. Left supramarginal gyrus

1-42. Damage to which region caused Morris's inability to tell right from left, and his inability to write, even with his nondominant hand?

a. Left parietal
b. Left frontal
c. Right frontal
d. Left temporal
e. Right temporal

1-43. A 10-month-old baby is being evaluated for visual problems and motor incoordination. Examination of this child's fundus reveals a bright "cherry-red spot" at the macula. Talking to the family of this visually impaired 10-month-old infant, you find that they are Jewish and their family is from the eastern portion of Europe (Ashkenazi Jews). Based on this specific family history, which one of the following enzymes is most likely to be deficient in this infant?

a. Aryl sulfatase
b. Beta-glucocerebrosidase
c. Hexosaminidase A
d. Hexosaminidase B
e. Sphingomyelinase

1-44. A 30-year-old secretary who is a single mother with two preschool children has frequent symptoms of generalized anxiety, tension, headaches, and insomnia. Which of the following behavioral interventions could be the most effective in relieving her symptoms?

a. Progressive muscle relaxation
b. Psychoanalysis
c. Hypnosis
d. Selective biofeedback
e. General psychotherapy

1-45. An 8-month-old infant is being evaluated for growth and mental retardation. Physical examination reveals a small infant with dry, rough skin, a protuberant abdomen, periorbital edema, a flattened, broad nose, and a large, protuberant tongue. Which one of the listed disorders is the most likely cause of this infant's signs and symptoms?

a. Graves' disease
b. Cretinism
c. Toxic multinodular goiter
d. Toxic adenoma
e. Struma ovarii

1-46. A 19-year-old male living in New Mexico presents to a local clinic after a one-day history of fever, myalgia, chills, headache, and malaise. He complains of vomiting, diarrhea, abdominal pain, tachypnea, and a productive cough. His white cell count was elevated with an increase in the number of bands. Atypical lymphocytes were also found in the peripheral blood. He was treated with antibiotics, but the next day he developed acute respiratory failure with cardiopulmonary arrest and died. Postmortem examination of the lungs revealed intraalveolar edema, rare hyaline membranes, and a few interstitial lymphoid aggregates. The most likely cause of this patient's illness is infection with

a.   Ebola virus
b.   Dengue fever virus
c.   Hanta virus
d.   Yellow fever virus
e.   Alpha virus

1-47. A 31-year-old female has been treated with fluoxetine for two months with no improvement in her depression. You decide to switch antidepressant therapy to phenelzine and instruct her to wait one week after stopping fluoxetine to start taking the new pills. She does not follow these instructions. Two days later, she is brought to the ED with unstable vital signs, muscle rigidity, myoclonus, and hyperthermia. What caused these findings?

a.   Increased serotonin (5-HT) in synapses
b.   Increased norepinephrine in synapses
c.   Increased acetylcholine in synapses
d.   Increased dopamine in synapses

1-48. A 55-year-old man who is being treated for adenocarcinoma of the lung is admitted to a hospital because of a temperature of 38.9°C (102°F), chest pain, and a dry cough. Sputum is collected. Gram's stain of the sputum is unremarkable and culture reveals many small gram negative rods able to grow only on a charcoal yeast extract agar. This organism most likely is

a.   *Klebsiella pneumoniae*
b.   *Mycoplasma pneumoniae*
c.   *Legionella pneumophila*
d.   *Chlamydia trachomatis*
e.   *Staphylococcus aureus*

1-49. A 49-year-old female presents with increasing problems swallowing food (progressive dysphagia). X-ray studies with contrast reveal that she has a markedly dilated esophagus above the level of the lower esophageal sphincter (LES). No lesions are seen within the lumen of the esophagus. This patient's symptoms are most likely caused by

a. Decreased LES resting pressure
b. Absence of myenteric plexus in the body of esophagus
c. Absence of myenteric plexus at the LES
d. Absence of submucosal plexus in the body of esophagus
e. Absence of submucosal plexus at the LES

1-50. A 19-year-old pregnant woman has a blood clot in her leg. Which of the following coagulation factors is not increased in pregnancy?

a. Factor VII
b. Factor VIII
c. Factor IX
d. Factor X
e. Factor XI

BLOCK 2

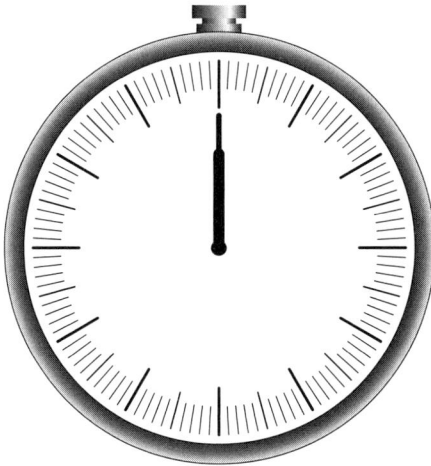

**YOU HAVE *60* MINUTES
TO COMPLETE *50* QUESTIONS.**

BLOCK 2

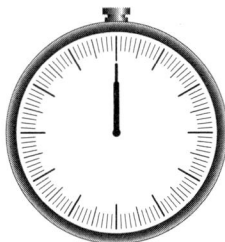

YOU HAVE **60** MINUTES
TO COMPLETE **50** QUESTIONS.

Questions

2-1. A 45-year-old male with alcoholic cirrhosis is seen in the ED because of a laceration of the scalp. Of the following local anesthetics, which would potentially be toxic?

a. Lidocaine
b. Benzocaine
c. Procaine
d. Tetracaine

2-2. A 35-year-old male who presents with a neck mass is found to have a serum calcium level of 11.8 mg/dL and periodic elevation of his blood pressure. Extensive work-up reveals the presence of a medullary carcinoma of the thyroid, a pheochromocytoma, and hyperplasia of the parathyroid glands. This patient most likely has

a. Multiple endocrine neoplasia syndrome (MEN) type I
b. MEN syndrome type IIa
c. MEN syndrome type IIb
d. Polyglandular syndrome type I
e. Polyglandular syndrome type II

2-3. A 6-year-old boy developed a facial rash that had the appearance of a slap to the face. The rash, which was composed of small red spots, subsequently involved the upper and lower extremities. The patient also complained of arthralgia and suddenly developed a life-threatening aplastic crisis of the bone marrow. The most likely infectious agent causing these symptoms is

a. Rhinovirus
b. Parainfluenza virus
c. Parvovirus
d. Measles virus
e. Rubella virus

2-4. A 48-year-old nurse develops clinical symptoms consistent with hepatitis. She recalls sticking herself with a needle approximately 4 months ago after drawing blood from a patient. Serologic tests for HBsAg, antibodies to HBsAg, and hepatitis A virus (HAV) are all negative; however, she is positive for IgM core antibody. The nurse

a. Does not have hepatitis B
b. Has hepatitis A
c. Is in the late stages of hepatitis B infection
d. Is in the "window" (after the disappearance of HBsAg and before the appearance of anti-HBsAg)
e. Has hepatitis C

2-5. A 5-year-old girl is brought to your office by her mother, who states that the girl has been drinking a lot of water lately. Your physical examination reveals a young girl whose eyes protrude slightly. Further work-up reveals the presence of multiple lytic bone lesions involving her calvarium and the base of her skull. What is the most likely diagnosis for this young girl?

a. Letterer-Siwe disease
b. Hand-Schuller-Christian disease
c. Dermatopathic lymphadenopathy
d. Unifocal Langerhans cell histiocytosis
e. Sarcoidosis

Clinical Case (Questions 2-6 through 2-9)

A 17-year-old high school football player presented to a neurology clinic because his mother thought that he may have acquired neck problems during a game. A month before, he had sustained a concussion from a blow to his head from another player. Shortly after, she noted that he intermittently tilted his head to the side. When asked what was the matter, he simply said that sometimes he had double vision, and that the images were situated on top of each other vertically, making it difficult to go down stairs. When examined, there was no neck pain or limitation of motion. He tended to keep his head tilted to the right side. When asked to follow the doctor's finger with his head in a straight position, his left eye would not move downward when his eyes were turned to the right, and tended to remain slightly deviated toward the left. At this point, he stated that he had double vision, and felt better if his head was tilted to the right. The remainder of his eye movements, as well as the remainder of his exam was normal.

2-6. Where has the damage occurred?

a. The oculomotor nerve
b. The abducens nerve
c. The trochlear nerve
d. The trigeminal nerve
e. The facial nerve

2-7. Which muscle is weakened?

a. Superior rectus
b. Inferior rectus
c. Lateral rectus
d. Superior oblique
e. Inferior oblique

2-8. From which portion of the brainstem has the damaged nerve emerged?

a. Right ventral midbrain
b. Right dorsal midbrain
c. Left ventral midbrain
d. Left dorsal midbrain
e. Left ventral pons

2-9. What is the action of the weak muscle?

a. Outward and upward rotation of the eye
b. Outward and downward rotation of the eye
c. Inward and upward rotation of the eye
d. Inward and downward rotation of the eye
e. Deviation of the eye laterally

2-10. A 49-year-old male presents with symptoms that developed following a long weekend of binge drinking. His serum reveals a gamma-glutamyl transferase (GGT) level of 65 IU/L. A liver biopsy reveals fatty change (steatosis) of numerous hepatocytes. This patient's liver abnormality is most likely the result of

a. Decreased free fatty acid delivery to the liver
b. Decreased production of triglycerides
c. Increased mitochondrial oxidation of fatty acids
d. Increased NADH production
e. Increased release of lipoproteins

2-11. A newborn female is being worked up clinically for several congenital abnormalities. During this work-up, it is discovered that the normal development of the vagina and uterus in this female infant had not occurred. Failure of the uterus to develop (agenesis) is directly related to the failure of what embryonic structure to develop?

a. Urogenital ridge
b. Mesonephric duct
c. Paramesonephric duct
d. Metanephric duct
e. Epoophoron

2-12. A 35-year-old European male, who is an avid beer drinker, presents with the sudden onset of signs of heart failure. If these symptoms are the result of cobalt put in his beer as a foam stabilizer, then gross examination of this patient's heart would most likely reveal

a. No gross abnormalities
b. Four chamber dilation with hypertrophy
c. Asymmetric septal hypertrophy
d. A stiff, hypocontracting heart
e. Constrictive cardiomyopathy

2-13. A known alcoholic is brought to the emergency room following an altercation in a local bar. The intern observes respiratory irregularity, coma, and papilledema. Emergency surgery is planned in order to prevent all the following EXCEPT

a. Brainstem herniation
b. Cerebellar herniation
c. Duret hemorrhages
d. Ruptured aneurysm
e. Death of the patient

2-14. A 9-year-old boy suddenly develops severe testicular pain. He is taken to the emergency room where he is evaluated and immediately taken to surgery. There his left testis is found to be markedly hemorrhagic due to testicular torsion. This abnormality caused a hemorrhagic testicular infarction because of

a. Arterial occlusion
b. Septic infarction
c. The collateral blood supply of the testis
d. The dual blood supply of the testis
e. Venous occlusion

2-15. A 26-year-old female with acquired immunodeficiency syndrome (AIDS) develops cryptococcal meningitis. She refuses all intravenous (IV) medication. Which antifungal agent can be given orally to treat the meningeal infection?

a. Ketoconazole
b. Amphotericin B
c. Fluconazole
d. Nystatin

2-16. A full-term male infant displays projectile vomiting 1 h after suckling. There is failure to gain weight during the first 2 weeks. The vomitus is not bile-stained and no respiratory difficulty is evident. Examination reveals an abdomen neither tense nor bloated. The most probable explanation is

a. Congenital hypertrophic pyloric stenosis
b. Duodenal atresia
c. Patent ileal diverticulum
d. Imperforate anus
e. Tracheoesophageal fistula

2-17. A 25-year-old female presents with fever, malaise, headaches, and muscle pain (myalgia). A chest x-ray reveals bilateral infiltrates. You draw a tube of blood in this patient (the tube contains anticoagulant) and place the tube in a cup of ice. After the blood has cooled, you notice that the red cells have agglutinated (not clotted). This agglutination goes away after you warm up the tube of blood. This patient's illness is most likely due to infection with

a. Influenza A virus
b. *Mycoplasma pneumonia*
c. *Streptococcal pneumonia*
d. *Pneumocystis pneumonia*
e. *Mycobacteria tuberculosis*

2-18. A 20-year-old man has headaches, blurred vision, and lateralizing neurologic deficits. An intracranial mass lesion is found. Microbial etiologies would include all of the following EXCEPT

a. *Aspergillus*
b. *Toxoplasma gondii*
c. *Bacteroides* spp.
d. *Escherichia coli*

2-19. A 42-year-old female patient delays initiation of movement, displays an uneven trajectory in moving her hand from above her head to touch her nose, and is uneven in her attempts to demonstrate rapid alternation of pronating and supernating movements of the hand and forearm. She probably has a lesion in the

a. Hemispheres of the posterior cerebellar lobe
b. Flocculonodular lobe of the cerebellum
c. Vermal region of the anterior cerebellar lobe
d. Fastigial nucleus
e. Ventral spinocerebellar tract

2-20. A 34-year-old male presents with multiple large, sharply defined, silver-white scaly plaques on the extensor surfaces of his elbows, knees, and scalp. Physical examination reveals discoloration and pitting of his fingernails. Lifting of one of the scales on his elbows produces multiple, minute areas of bleeding (positive Auspitz sign). Histologic sections from one of the scaly plaques would most likely reveal

a. Subepithelial bullae
b. Regular elongation of the rete ridges
c. Liquefactive degeneration of the basal layer of the epidermis
d. Increased granular cell layer
e. Chronic inflammation below a zone of degenerated collagen

2-21. A 45-year-old male presents with severe pain in both knee joints. At the time of surgery, his cartilage is found to have a dark blue-black color. Further evaluation revealed that this patient's urine darkened rapidly with time. The most likely diagnosis for this abnormality is

a. Hyperphenylalaninemia
b. Tyrosinemia
c. Tyrosinase-positive oculocutaneous albinism
d. Alcaptonuria
e. Maple syrup urine disease

2-22. A 40-year-old male is HIV-positive with a cluster of differentiation 4 (CD4) count of 200/mm^3. Within two months, he develops a peripheral white blood cell count of 1000/mm^3 and a hemoglobin of 9.0 mg/dL. Which drug has most likely caused the adverse effect?

a. Acyclovir
b. Dideoxycytidine
c. Foscarnet
d. Rimantadine
e. Zidovudine

Clinical Case (Questions 2-23 through 2-26)

Audrey is a 45-year-old woman who was brought to her local hospital's emergency room by her husband because of several days of progressive weakness and numbness in her arms and legs. Her symptoms had begun with tingling in her toes, which she assumed to be her feet "falling asleep." However, this feeling did not disappear, and she began to feel numb, first in her toes on both feet, then ascending to her calves and knees. Two days later, Audrey began to feel numb in her fingertips and had difficulty lifting her legs. When she finally was unable to climb the stairs of her house because of her leg weakness, difficulty gripping the banister, and shortness of breath, her husband urged her to go to the emergency room.

The neurologist who examined Audrey in the emergency room noticed that she was short of breath while sitting in bed. He asked the respiratory therapist to measure her vital capacity (the greatest volume of air that can be exhaled from the lungs after a maximal inspiration), and the value for this was far lower than was expected for her age and weight. Her neurologic examination showed that her arms and legs were very weak, so that she had difficulty lifting them against gravity. She was unable to feel a pin or a vibrating tuning fork at all on her legs and below her elbows, but was able to feel the pin on her upper chest. The neurologist could not elicit any reflexes from her ankles or knees. He subsequently advised the emergency room staff that Audrey needed to have a spinal tap, and be admitted to the intensive care unit immediately.

2-23. Where in the nervous system is the damage?

a. Frontal lobe
b. Temporal lobe
c. Peripheral nerves and nerve roots
d. Spinal cord
e. Muscle

2-24. Audrey can't feel a pinprick in certain locations. Which receptor carries this information?

a. Merkel disc
b. Ruffini corpuscle
c. Pacinian corpuscle
d. C- and A-delta fibers
e. Meissner

2-25. Which receptor should be activated by the tuning fork?

a. C- and A-delta fibers
b. Merkel
c. Pacinian
d. Ruffini
e. Meissner

2-26. The absent reflexes are a sign of a lesion of which portion of the nervous system?

a. The frontal lobe
b. The dorsal horn of the spinal cord or any point distal to this structure
c. Brainstem
d. Cervical corticospinal tract
e. Any point proximal to the upper cervical spinal cord

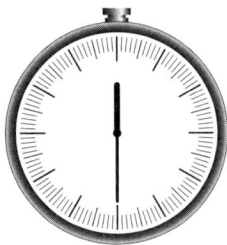

YOU SHOULD HAVE COMPLETED APPROXIMATELY
25 QUESTIONS AND HAVE 30 MINUTES REMAINING.

2-27. Based on physical findings, you suspect that a 48-year-old woman has acromegaly. The definitive diagnostic test for acromegaly is measurement of growth hormone in the following setting:

a. Random
b. Thyrotropin-releasing hormone (TRH) stimulation test
c. Insulin tolerance test
d. Oral glucose tolerance test
e. Luteinizing hormone-releasing hormone (LHRH) stimulation test

2-28. A child with cleft palate, a heart defect, and extra fifth fingers is found to have 46 chromosomes with extra material on one homologue of the chromosome 5 pair. This chromosomal abnormality is best described by which of the following terms?

a. Polyploidy
b. Balanced rearrangement
c. Ring formation
d. Mosaicism
e. Unbalanced rearrangement

2-29. A 59-year-old male is found to have a 3.5 cm mass in the right upper lobe of his lung. A biopsy of this mass is diagnosed as a moderately differentiated squamous cell carcinoma. Work-up reveals that no bone metastases are present, but laboratory examination reveals that his serum calcium levels are 11.5 mg/dL. This patient's paraneoplastic syndrome is most likely the result of production of

a. Parathyroid hormone
b. Parathyroid hormone-related peptide
c. Calcitonin
d. Calcitonin-related peptide
e. Erythropoietin

2-30. A 66-year-old man with no previous significant illness presents with back pain. The patient had felt well except for an increase in fatigue over the past few months. He suddenly felt severe low back pain while raising his garage door. Physical examination reveals a well-developed white male in acute pain. His pulse is 88 beats per minute and blood pressure is 150/90 mmHg. The conjunctivae are pale. There is marked tenderness to percussion over the lumbar spine. The following laboratory data are obtained: hemoglobin 11.0 g/dL (normal 13 to 16 g/dL), serum calcium 12.3 mg/dL (normal 8.5 to 11 mg/dL), abnormal serum protein electrophoresis with a monoclonal IgG spike, urine positive for Bence Jones protein, abnormal plasma cells in bone marrow. X-rays reveal lytic lesions of the skull and pelvis and a compression fracture of lumbar vertebrae.

Your diagnosis would be

a. Osteoporosis
b. Osteomalacia
c. Multiple myeloma
d. Hypoparathyroidism
e. Paget's disease

2-31. A 49-year-old female presents with increasing fatigue and is found to have elevated liver enzymes (AST and ALT). You follow her in your clinical and find over the next nine months that her liver enzymes have remained elevated. All serologic tests for viral markers are within normal limits. A liver biopsy reveals chronic inflammation in the portal triads that focally destroys the limiting plate and "spills over" into the adjacent hepatocytes. There are no granulomas present, and there is no evidence of fibrosis surrounding any of the bile ducts within the portal triads. Antismooth muscle antibodies and antinuclear antibodies are found in her serum. An LE cell test is positive. What is the diagnosis?

a. Autoimmune hepatitis
b. Chronic persistent hepatitis
c. Primary biliary cirrhosis
d. Primary sclerosing cholangitis
e. Systemic lupus erythematosus

2-32. A 28-year-old man is treated in an emergency room for a superficial gash on his forehead. The wound is bleeding profusely, but examination reveals no fracture. While the wound is being sutured, he relates that while he was using an electric razor, he remembers becoming dizzy and then "waking up on the floor with blood everywhere." The physician suspects a hypersensitive cardiac reflex.

Which of the following statements best characterizes the carotid reflex?

a. It is normally initiated in the carotid body by changes in the partial pressures of oxygen
b. It is normally initiated in the carotid sinus by changes in arterial pressure
c. The associated nerve pathways lie external to the carotid sheath
d. The sensory receptors are located in the vicinity of the aortic arch

2-33. Mr. Baker, a 40-year-old stockbroker, is stressed and worried because he feels he has many of the personality and physical character-istics which place him at risk for coronary heart disease. His physical examination, laboratory results, symptoms, and electrocardiogram tapes confirm that he is indeed at moderate risk for a coronary. To assess which of his personality and behavioral patterns could put him at an even higher risk for a coro-nary, it would be best to test him with the

a. Millon Behavioral Health Inventory
b. Cohen Perceived Stress Scale
c. Rosenman and Friedman Type A Structured Interview
d. Jenkins Activity Survey of Type A Behavior
e. Cook-Medley Hostility Inventory

2-34. A 36-year-old male heroin addict is seen in the ED because he cannot be aroused from sleep. On examination, he has shallow breathing and pinpoint pupils. Naloxone is administered, and the patient wakes up. Which of the opi-ate receptor subtypes that binds naloxone is responsible for revers-ing the respiratory depression and miosis?

a. δ
b. κ
c. μ

2-35. A 28-year-old male bitten by a bee is rushed into the emergency room with a variety of symptoms including increasing difficulty in breathing due to vasal and bron-chial construction. While your sub-sequent treatment is to block the effects of histamine and other acute-acting biochemicals released by most cells, you also must block the slow-reacting substance of anaphy-laxis (SRS-A), which is the most potent constrictor of the muscles enveloping the bronchial passages. What is SRS-A composed of?

a. Thromboxanes
b. Interleukins
c. Complement
d. Leukotrienes
e. Prostaglandins

2-36. Ten minutes after being stung by a wasp, a 30-year-old male develops multiple patches of red, irregular skin lesions over his entire body. These lesions (urticaria) are pruritic, and new crops of lesions occur every day. This response is primarily the result of liberation of specific vasoactive substances by the action of

a. Activated T lymphocytes on smooth muscle cells
b. IgA on basophils and mast cells
c. IgA on lymphocytes and eosinophils
d. IgE on basophils and mast cells
e. IgE on lymphocytes and eosinophils

2-37. A perimenopausal woman presents with increasing swallowing difficulty and fatigue. Physical examination reveals that her thyroid is enlarged (palpable goiter). Laboratory examination of her serum reveals T_4 of 4.9 μg/dL, free T_4 of 2.5 ng/dL, and TSH levels of 5.5 μIU/mL. No thyroid-stimulating immunoglobulins are identified in the serum, but anti-microsomal antibodies are present. Examination of histologic section from her thyroid gland reveals numerous lymphocytes, some forming lymphoid follicles, and atrophy of the thyroid follicles with focal oxyphilic metaplasia. The most likely diagnosis is

a. Hashimoto's thyroiditis
b. DeQuervain's thyroiditis
c. Subacute lymphocytic thyroiditis
d. Riedel's thyroiditis
e. Thyrotoxicosis

2-38. A child comes to an emergency room because of an infected dog bite. The wound is found to contain small Gram-negative rods. The most likely cause of infection is

a. *Escherichia coli*
b. *Haemophilus influenzae*
c. *Pasteurella multocida*
d. *Brucella canis*
e. *Klebsiella rhinoscleromatis*

2-39. Several days after exploring a new cave in eastern Kentucky, a 39-year-old female develops shortness of breath and a low-grade fever. Chest x-rays reveal several irregular areas in both upper lung fields along with enlarged hilar and mediastinal lymph nodes. A biopsy of one of these lymph nodes reveals granulomatous inflammation. Multiple small yeast surrounded by clear zones are seen within macrophages. Which one of the following organisms is most likely responsible for this individual's disease?

a. *Aspergillus* species
b. *Blastomyces dermatitidis*
c. *Candida albicans*
d. *Histoplasma capsulatum*
e. *Mucor*

Clinical Case (Questions 2-40 through 2-43)

John is a 57-year-old man who has always been a very heavy drinker, often consuming two pints of whiskey per day, for many years. Upon the urging of his wife, he decided to seek medical attention for help with problems with his gait, which has steadily worsened over the past several months. He noticed that he now needed to stand with his feet far apart in order to maintain his balance, and "waddled" when he walked.

The doctor who evaluated him tested his memory and speech carefully, as well as his cranial nerves, and was unable to find any deficits. There was no weakness, sensory loss, or abnormalities in his reflexes. When asked to touch the doctor's finger, then his nose, John missed his nose slightly, but rapidly corrected the movement on both sides. When asked to slide his right heel down his left shin, his heel slid sideways and clumsily across the bone until it reached his ankle. The response with the left heel was similar. When asked to walk, John walked with his feet very far apart. If he attempted to walk in a tandem fashion, with one heel in front of the other toe, he began to fall, and the doctor needed to catch him. The doctor ordered an MRI (magnetic resonance imaging) of John's head.

2-40. What term could one use for John's gait?

a. Stiff
b. Festinating
c. Ataxic
d. Spastic
e. Shuffling

2-41. A gait problem of this type could be caused by lesions in which system(s)?

a. Cerebellar tracts only
b. Posterior columns only
c. Corticospinal tracts
d. Both the cerebellar and posterior column systems
e. Spinothalamic system

2-42. Where in the brain would a neurologist expect to visualize the lesion on a magnetic resonance image scan (MRI scan)?

a. Red nucleus
b. Cerebellar vermis
c. Substantia nigra
d. Internal capsule
e. Basilar pons

2-43. The region of the affected area is associated with which functional division of the cerebellum?

a. Cerebrocerebellum
b. Spinocerebellum
c. Dentate nucleus
d. Brachium conjunctivum
e. Brachium pontis

2-44. A 45-year-old man presents with weakness and cramping that involves both of his hands. Physical examination reveals atrophy of the muscles of both hands, hyperactive reflexes and muscle fasciculations involving his arms and legs, and a positive Babinski reflex. Sensation appears normal in his arms and legs. The most likely diagnosis for this individual is

a.   Metachromatic leukodystrophy
b.   Amyotrophic lateral sclerosis
c.   Guillain-Barré syndrome
d.   Huntington disease
e.   Wilson disease

2-45. An 28-year-old anemic female is found to have hypochromic, microcytic red cells. Additional tests reveal the serum iron levels, the total iron-binding capacity, and the transferrin saturation to all be reduced. A bone marrow biopsy reveals the iron to be present mainly within macrophages. The most likely diagnosis is

a.   Iron deficiency
b.   Thalassemia trait
c.   Anemia of chronic disease
d.   Sideroblastic anemia
e.   Pernicious anemia

2-46. A 2-year-old girl is being evaluated from marked swelling of her neck. During the work-up of this patient, a karyotype reveals that she is monosomic for the X chromosome. Which one of the listed abnormalities is most likely responsible for the swelling of this young girl's neck?

a.   Bacillary angiomatosis
b.   Capillary hemangioma
c.   Cystic hygroma
d.   Glomus tumor
e.   Spider angioma

2-47. A 39-year-old male who has the autosomal dominant gene for type I osteogenesis imperfecta has blue scleras and slightly reduced height, whereas his brother has multiple fractures and deformities. This is an example of

a.   Polymorphism
b.   Mutation
c.   Variable expressivity
d.   Fitness

2-48. A 30-year-old man presents with weight gain, dorsocervical fat pad, and proximal muscle weakness. His urinary free cortisol level is markedly elevated and does not suppress with dexamethasone. The plasma ACTH is undetectable. Your best next diagnostic test is

a. Serum antidiuretic hormone (ADH)
b. Chest CT
c. MRI of the pituitary
d. ACTH stimulation test
e. Abdominal CT

2-49. A 36-year-old male unemployed dishwasher with no history of seizures presents with difficulty thinking coherently and claiming he is an astronaut. Following treatment, he suddenly has a grand mal seizure. Which neuroleptic agent was administered?

a. Haloperidol
b. Fluphenazine
c. Clozapine
d. Molindone
e. Loxapine

2-50. A 45-year-old male alcoholic vomits blood and is hypotensive. The most likely cause of his bleeding episode is related to

a. Achalasia
b. Plummer-Vinson syndrome
c. Sliding hiatal hernia
d. Zenker's diverticula
e. Esophageal varices

BLOCK 3

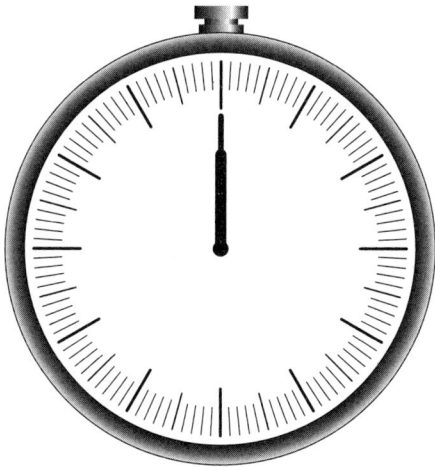

YOU HAVE **60** MINUTES
TO COMPLETE **50** QUESTIONS.

BLOCK 3

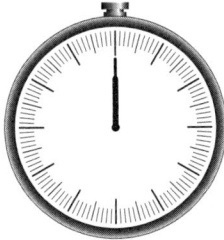

YOU HAVE *60* MINUTES
TO COMPLETE *50* QUESTIONS.

Questions

3-1. A 67-year-old woman slipped on a scatter rug and fell with her right arm extended in an attempt to ease the impact of the fall. She experienced immediate severe pain in the region of the right collar bone and in the right wrist. Painful movement of the right arm was minimized by holding the arm close to the body and by supporting the elbow with the left hand.

The frequency of clavicular fracture is best explained by the

a. Early beginning of ossification
· b. Late completion of ossification
c. S-shape of this bone
d. Strong articulation with the coracoid process
e. Subcutaneous location of the bone

3-2. An 11-year-old Jamaican boy develops a massive benign enlargement of the cervical lymph nodes associated with fever and leukocytosis. Which of the following lymph node disorders could account for these findings?

a. Toxoplasmosis
b. Histiocytic medullary reticulosis
c. Burkitt's disease
d. Sinus histiocytosis with massive lymphadenopathy (SHML)
e. Angioimmunoblastic lymphadenopathy with dysproteinemia

3-3. An 82-year-old male treated for congestive heart failure for years with digitalis and furosemide dies of pulmonary edema. A postmortem examination of the heart would most likely show

a. Severe left ventricular hypertrophy
b. Right and left ventricular hypertrophy
c. Right ventricular infarction
d. Aortic and mitral valve stenosis
e. A dilated, globular heart with thin walls

3-4. A 65-year-old male presents with bone pain and is found to have hypocalcemia and increased parathyroid hormone. Surgical exploration of his neck finds all four of his parathyroid glands to be enlarged. Without any other information, which one of the following is most likely the cause of the enlargement of the parathyroid glands?

a. Primary hyperplasia
b. Parathyroid adenoma
c. Chronic renal failure
d. Parathyroid carcinoma
e. Lung carcinoma

3-5. A 40-year-old man has erectile dysfunction. He is noted to have hyperprolactinemia (prolactin of 400 µg/L). On MRI, a macroadenoma with superstellar extension is found. The best course of therapy for the patient is

a. Medical therapy with bromocriptine
b. Transsphenoidal surgery
c. Transfrontal surgery
d. Medical therapy with somatostatin agonist
e. Thyroxine

3-6. A 28-year-old menstruating woman appeared in the emergency room with the following signs and symptoms: fever, 104°F (40°C); WBC, 16,000/mm³; blood pressure, 90/65 mmHg; a scarlatiniform rash on her trunk, palms, and soles; extreme fatigue; vomiting; and diarrhea.

The patient described in the case above most likely has

a. Scalded skin syndrome
b. Toxic shock syndrome
c. Guillain-Barré syndrome
d. Chickenpox
e. Staphylococcal food poisoning

Clinical Case (Questions 3-7 through 3-10)
Lindsey is a 12-year-old girl who has never had medical problems. One day, while in the kitchen with her mother, she told her mother that she felt very frightened all of a sudden, and had a funny feeling in her stomach. Immediately after this, she turned her head to the right, stared persistently, and began to chew. Her mother called her name several times, but Lindsey, who was usually a very obedient child, did not answer. After approximately one minute of staring, Lindsey slowly turned her head back to her mother. Apparently confused, she asked her mother where she was. Over the next 10 to 15 minutes, she became less and less confused, and by the time she was in the car being driven to the pediatrician by her mother, she felt like she was back to normal.

The pediatrician listened to Lindsey's mother's story when they arrived. He examined Lindsey, and could find no abnormalities on general physical examination, or on neurologic examination. The pediatrician told her mother that he would refer Lindsey to a pediatric neurologist for further evaluation, as well as further evaluation for the need for medication.

3-7. What type of problem did Lindsey most likely have?

a. Attention deficit disorder
b. Temporary psychosis
c. Conversion disorder
d. Epilepsy
e. Schizophrenia

3-8. From which area of the brain is this problem most likely emanating?

a. Medulla
b. Occipital lobe
c. Temporal lobe
d. Thalamus
e. Midbrain

3-9. If the amygdala is involved with this problem, which two major efferent pathways from this structure may be effected?

a. Corticospinal tract and stria terminalis
b. Mamillothalamic tract and stria terminalis
c. Medial forebrain bundle and stria terminalis
d. Ventral amygdalofugal pathway and stria terminalis
e. Corticospinal tract and mamillothalamic tract

3-10. If the hippocampal formation is involved in this problem, which structures may be damaged?

a. Hippocampus, dentate gyrus, and subiculum
b. Hippocampus, amygdala, and subiculum
c. Hippocampus, fornix, and amygdala
d. Hippocampus, fornix, and habenulae
e. Hippocampus, dentate gyrus, and fornix

3-11. A 48-year-old male who has a long history of excessive drinking presents with signs of alcoholic hepatitis. Microscopic examination of a biopsy of this patient's liver reveals irregular eosinophilic hyaline inclusions within the cytoplasm of the hepatocytes. These eosinophilic inclusions are composed of

a. Immunoglobulin
b. Excess plasma proteins
c. Prekeratin intermediate filaments
d. Basement membrane material
e. Lipofuscin

3-12. A 30-year-old male with a two-year history of chronic renal failure requiring dialysis consents to transplantation. A donor kidney becomes available. He is given cyclosporine to prevent transplant rejection just before surgery. What is the most likely adverse effect of this drug?

a. Bone marrow depression
b. Nephrotoxicity
c. Oral and GI ulceration
d. Pancreatitis
e. Seizures

3-13. A 24-year-old male has an autosomal dominantly inherited disease. The patient and his grandfather show evidence of disease, but the patient's father is asymptomatic. This is an example of

a. Polymorphism
b. Mutation
c. Variable expressivity
d. Reduced penetrance

3-14. A 17-year-old high school student died suddenly while playing basketball. At autopsy asymmetric hypertrophy of the interventricular septum was discovered. Histologic sections from this area revealed disorganization of the myofibers, which were thicker than normal and had hyperchromatic nuclei. What is the most likely diagnosis?

a. Hypertrophic cardiomyopathy
b. Dilated cardiomyopathy
c. Constrictive cardiomyopathy
d. Secondary cardiomyopathy
e. Endomyocardial fibrosis

3-15. A 52-year-old female presents with nausea, fatigue, muscle weakness, and intermittent pain in her left flank. Laboratory examination reveals an increased serum calcium and a decreased serum phosphorus. Her plasma parathyroid hormone levels are increased, but parathyroid hormone-related peptide levels are within normal limits. Urinary calcium is increased, and microhematuria is present. Her abnormality is most likely caused by

a. Primary hyperparathyroidism
b. Primary hypoparathyroidism
c. Pseudohypoparathyroidism
d. Secondary hyperparathyroidism
e. Secondary hypoparathyroidism

3-16. A 41-year-old male presents with involuntary rapid jerky movements and progressive dementia. He soon dies and gross examination of his brain reveals marked degeneration of the caudate nucleus. This individual's symptoms were caused by

a. Decreased functioning of GABA neurons
b. Increased functioning of dopamine neurons
c. Relative increased functioning of acetylcholine neurons
d. Relative decreased functioning of acetylcholine neurons
e. Decreased functioning of serotonin neurons

3-17. A 38-year-old woman has had amenorrhea for 6 months, with increased cold intolerance, loss of energy, and hair loss. Her menses were normal until this episode started, and she has also gained 22 pounds over these 6 months. Her pregnancy test is negative. Which test would you now order?

a. FSH and LH levels
b. Estrogen level
c. Testosterone level
d. TSH level
e. Cortisol level

3-18. An apathetic male infant in an underdeveloped country is found to have peripheral edema, a "moon" face, and an enlarged, fatty liver. Which of the following is one mechanism involved in the pathogenesis of this child's abnormalities?

a. Decreased protein intake leading to decreased lipoproteins
b. Decreased caloric intake leading to hypoalbuminemia
c. Decreased carbohydrate intake leading to hypoglycemia
d. Decreased fluid intake leading to hypernatremia
e. Decreased fat absorption leading to hypovitaminosis

3-19. A 32-year-old female presents with the recent onset of oligomenorrhea followed by amenorrhea, and then the loss of female secondary characteristics. She has also developed acne, deepening of her voice, and temporal balding. Which one of the following ovarian tumors would most likely produce these symptoms?

a. Epithelial tumor
b. Stromal tumor
c. Germ cell tumor
d. Surface tumor
e. Metastasis

3-20. A 31-year-old female is treated with an antipsychotic agent because of a recent history of spontaneously removing her clothing in public places and claiming that she hears voices telling her to do so. Her blood pressure is normally 130/70 mmHg. Since being treated with a drug, she has had several bouts of syncope. Orthostatic hypotension was noted on physical examination. Which drug is most likely to cause this?

a. Haloperidol
b. Molindone
c. Loxapine
d. Thioridazine
e. Pimozide

3-21. A 4-year-old boy presents to the physician's office with coarse facies, short stature, stiffening of the joints, and mental retardation. Both parents, a 10-year-old sister, and an 8-year-old brother all appear unaffected. The patient's mother is pregnant. She also had a brother who died at 15 years of age with similar findings that seemed to worsen with age. She also has a nephew (her sister's son) who exhibits similar features. You suspect a diagnosis of Hunter syndrome.

The most likely pattern of inheritance for this condition is

a. Autosomal dominant
b. Autosomal recessive
c. X-linked dominant
d. X-linked recessive
e. None of the above

3-22. An 18-year-old African-American woman comes to your medical clinic with enlarged, fixed, hardened, and matted lymph nodes in her neck. She denies weight loss, fevers, and night sweats. The etiology of this abnormality includes all EXCEPT

a. Periodontal abscess
b. Thyroid cysts
c. Infection in a salivary gland
d. *Pseudomonas* spp.

3-23. A 38-year-old woman presents with fatigue and pruritus and is found to have high serum alkaline phosphatase and slightly elevated serum bilirubin levels. Serum antimitochondrial antibodies are also present. A liver biopsy reveals a marked lymphocytic infiltrate in the portal tracts along with occasional granulomas. The most likely diagnosis is

a. Impacted gallstone
b. Primary biliary cirrhosis
c. Primary sclerosing cholangitis
d. Von Meyenburg's complex
e. Caroli's disease

3-24. Following a diet fad meal of skim milk and yogurt, an 35-year-old female experiences abdominal distention, nausea, cramping, and pain followed by a watery diarrhea. This set of symptoms has been observed each time the meal is consumed. A likely diagnosis is

a. Steatorrhea
b. Lactase deficiency
c. Maltose deficiency
d. Sialilase deficiency
e. Lipoprotein lipase deficiency

3-25. A 52-year-old male presents with symptoms of gastric pain after eating. While working up this patient, a 3-cm mass is found in the wall of the stomach. This mass is resected and histologic examination reveals a tumor composed of cells having elongated, spindle-shaped nuclei. The tumor does not connect to the overlying epithelium and is found only in the wall of the stomach. This tumor most likely originated from

a. Adipocytes
b. Endothelial cells
c. Glandular epithelial cells
d. Smooth muscle cells
e. Squamous epithelial cells

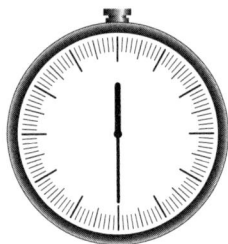

YOU SHOULD HAVE COMPLETED APPROXIMATELY
25 QUESTIONS AND HAVE 30 MINUTES REMAINING.

3-26. A woman who is 5 weeks post partum (normal delivery, healthy child) develops bleeding episodes with oliguria and hematuria. No fever or neurologic manifestations are present. The blood urea nitrogen level is 65 mg/dL; a peripheral blood smear is presented in the photomicrograph below. This patient most likely has

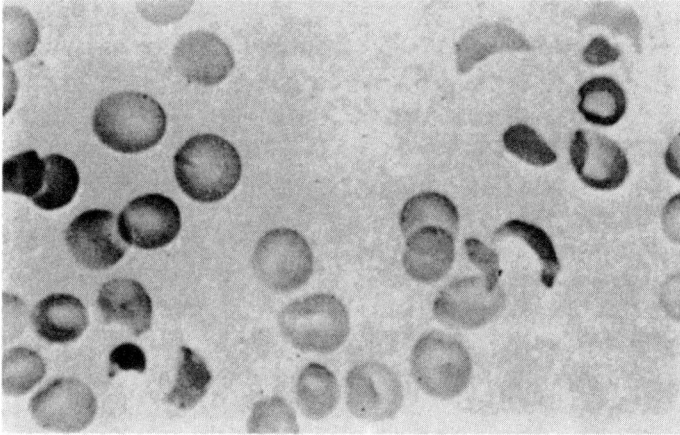

a. Thrombotic thrombocytopenic purpura
b. Autoimmune thrombocytopenic purpura
c. Hemolytic uremic syndrome
d. Disseminated intravascular coagulopathy
e. Sickle cell crisis

3-27. A 29-year-old male hospital worker is found to have hepatitis B surface antigen. Subsequent tests reveal the presence of *e* antigen as well. The worker most likely

a. Is infective and has active hepatitis
b. Is infective but does not have active hepatitis
c. Is not infective
d. Is evincing a biologic false positive test for hepatitis
e. Has both hepatitis B and C

3-28. A 74-year-old male has had trouble urinating for 1 week. The force of the urinary stream is reduced, but there is no difficulty starting the stream. There is no pain. What is the problem?

a. Decreased detrusor contractility
b. Detrusor instability
c. Detrusor failure
d. Acute urinary obstruction
e. Chronic urinary obstruction

3-29. A 2-month-old girl presents with a soft, high-pitched, mewing cry and is found to have several congenital heart defects. The most likely chromosomal abnormality producing these symptoms is

a. $5p^-$
b. $11p^-$
c. $13q^-$
d. $21q^-$
e. $22q^-$

3-30. A 29-year-old male requires suturing for a deep laceration in his palm. He is allergic to benzocaine. Which of the following local anesthetics could safely be used?

a. Cocaine
b. Tetracaine
c. Bupivacaine
d. Procaine

3-31. A 4-year-old male infant weighing seven pounds six ounces is brought to the emergency room by his parents. The examining ER physician notes that his skin and sclerae are icteric. A blood test indicates elevated bilirubin conjugated to glucuronic acid.

The elevated bilirubin levels in this patient are most likely the result of:

a. Deficiency of enzymes regulating bilirubin solubility
b. Hepatocellular proliferation
c. Decreased destruction of red blood cells
d. Dilation of the common bile duct
e. Increased hepatocyte uptake of bilirubin

3-32. A 61-year-old male presents with increasing shortness of breath. A chest x-ray reveals a diffuse pulmonary infiltrate, while a transbronchial biopsy reveals fibrosis of the walls of the alveoli, many of which contain sheets of "desquamated" cells. Which of the following would be the best therapy for this patient?

a. Theophylline
b. Steroids
c. Antibiotics
d. Isoniazid
e. Symptomatic treatment only

3-33. A 7-year-old girl presents with fever, abdominal pain, and painful joints (arthralgia). After taking a careful history you discover that she had a sore throat about two weeks prior to the onset of these signs and symptoms. If this young patient had developed a hypersensitivity vasculitis, then which one of the following skin lesions would be most indicative of cutaneous hemorrhage secondary to vasculitis?

a.   Petechiae
b.   Palpable purpura
c.   Nonpalpable purpura
d.   Ecchymoses
e.   Telangiectasis

3-34. A young girl has repeated infections with *Candida albicans* and respiratory viruses since the time she was 3 months old. As part of the clinical evaluation of her immune status, her responses to routine immunization procedures should be tested. In this evaluation, the use of which of the following vaccines is contraindicated?

a.   Diphtheria toxoid
b.   *Bordetella pertussis* vaccine
c.   Tetanus toxoid
d.   BCG
e.   Inactivated polio

3-35. A 19-year-old woman is diagnosed with tuberculosis (TB). Before prescribing a drug regimen, you take a careful medication history because one of the drugs commonly used to treat TB induces microsomal cytochrome P-450 enzymes in the liver. Which drug is this?

a.   Isoniazid
b.   Rifampin
c.   Pyrazinamide
d.   Ethambutol
e.   Vitamin B6

3-36. A 38-year-old male with AIDS presents with decreasing mental status. The work-up at this time includes a spinal tap. Cerebrospinal fluid (CSF) is stained with a mucicarmine stain and India ink. The mucicarmine stain reveals numerous yeast that stain bright red. The India ink prep reveals through negative staining that these yeast have a capsule. What is your diagnosis?

a.   Chromomycosis
b.   Coccidioidomycosis
c.   Cryptococcosis
d.   Cryptosporidiosis
e.   Paracoccidioidomycosis

3-37. A 25-year-old schoolteacher was well until she attended a church bazaar where she heartily ate barbecued turkey. The following day she developed bloody diarrhea, crampy pain, and tenesmus. A gastroenterologist who did not take a history took a colon biopsy specimen that showed mucosal edema, congestion, and numerous lymphoid cells in the lamina propria. Which of the following differential diagnoses would apply?

a. Staphylococcal gastroenteritis vs. Crohn's disease
b. Viral gastroenteritis vs. acute diverticulitis
c. Colonic endometriosis vs. amebic dysentery
d. Early ulcerative colitis vs. salmonella colitis
e. Bleeding hemorrhoids vs. Meckel's diverticulitis

3-38. A 54-year-old male presents with a wide-based, ataxic gait during his attempts at walking. He also is unsteady and sways when standing and displays a tendency to fall backward or to either side in a drunken manner. A lesion is most likely located in the

a. Hemispheres of the posterior cerebellar lobe
b. Anterior limb of the internal capsule
c. Dentate nucleus
d. Anterior lobe of the cerebellum
e. Flocculonodular lobe of the cerebellum

3-39. A 30-year-old male with recently developed AIDS is referred to you as a primary care physician. What is apt to be the most prominent psychosocial factor or reaction that you can expect and perhaps help prevent?

a. Loss of independence
b. Fear of losing confidentiality
c. Guilt
d. Depressed mood
e. Suicidal thoughts

3-40. After receiving incompatible blood, a 46-year-old male develops a transfusion reaction in the form of back pain, fever, shortness of breath, and hematuria. This type of immunologic reaction is classified as a

a. Systemic anaphylactic reaction
b. Systemic immune complex reaction
c. Delayed-type hypersensitivity reaction
d. Complement-mediated cytotoxicity
e. T-cell-mediated cytotoxicity

3-41. A 53-year-old banker develops paralysis on the right side of the face, which produces an expressionless and drooping appearance. He is unable to close the right eye and also has difficulty chewing and drinking. Examination shows loss of blink reflex in the right eye to stimulation of either right or left conjunctiva. Lacrimation appears normal on the right side, but salivation is diminished and taste is absent on the anterior right side of the tongue. There is no complaint of hyperacusis. Audition and balance appear to be normal. The lesion is located

a. In the brain and involves the nucleus of the facial nerve and superior salivatory nucleus
b. Within the internal auditory meatus
c. At the geniculate ganglion
d. In the facial canal just distal to the genu of the facial nerve
e. Just proximal to the stylomastoid foramen

3-42. You confirm acromegaly in a 58-year-old female, and an MRI of the pituitary shows a microadenoma. The best choice for treatment is

a. Transsphenoidal surgery
b. Medical therapy with somatostatin agonist
c. Irradiation
d. Medical therapy with bromocryptine
e. Transfrontal surgery

3-43. A 33-year-old female patient treated with haloperidol for a history of schizophrenia is seen in the ED because of complaints of fever, stiffness, and tremor. Her temperature is 104°F, and her serum creatine kinase (CK) level is elevated. What has occurred?

a. Overdose
b. Allergy
c. Neuroleptic malignant syndrome (NMS)
d. Tardive dyskinesia
e. Parkinsonism

3-44. A 75-year-old female presents with a pruritic vulvar lesion. Physical examination reveals an irregular white rough area involving her vulva. If this area of leukoplakia was due to lichen sclerosis, then biopsies from this area would most likely reveal

a. Atrophy of epidermis with dermal fibrosis
b. Epidermal atypia with dysplasia
c. Epithelial hyperplasia and hyperkeratosis
d. Individual malignant cells invading the epidermis
e. Loss of pigment in the epidermis

3-45. A 65-year-old male with a lung mass has increasing skin pigmentation and marked muscle weakness and wasting. His urinary free cortisol level is 690 μg/24 h (10 to 80) and is nonsuppressible. Which of the following laboratory tests would probably be most diagnostic?

a. ACTH stimulation test
b. MRI of the pituitary
c. CT of the abdomen
d. Plasma ACTH
e. Parathyroid hormone

3-46. During a routine breast self-examination, a 35-year-old female is concerned because her breasts feel "lumpy." She consults you as her primary care physician. After performing an examination, you reassure her that no masses are present, and that the "lumpiness" that she felt was due to fibrocystic changes. Considering this clinical opinion, a pathologic finding that is consistent with the nonproliferative form of fibrocystic change is

a. A blue-domed cyst
b. A radial scar
c. Atypical hyperplasia
d. Papillomatosis
e. Sclerosing adenosis

Clinical Case (Questions 3-47 through 3-50)

Bob is a 75-year-old male college graduate who was brought to a neurologist by his family because he was having problems with his gait, suffered from urinary incontinence for the past six months, and recently began to have problems with his short-term memory and paying his bills. The gait problem mainly manifested itself as difficulty in climbing stairs and frequent falls. Bob had no past medical history other than a subarachnoid hemorrhage resulting from a ruptured cerebral aneurysm many years earlier.

When the neurologist examined Bob, she found that he could not remember three objects five minutes after they were shown to him, even when he was prompted. He was unable to figure out how many quarters were in $1.75, and spelled the word "world" incorrectly. A grasp reflex (squeezing the examiner's hand as a reflex reaction to stroking of the palm) was present. Although his motor strength was full in all of his extremities, when asked to walk, he took many steps in the same place without moving forward, then started to fall. His cranial nerve, sensory, and cerebellar examinations were normal.

3-47. Bob has a grasp reflex and dementia. A lesion in which region can cause this deficit?

a. Occipital lobe
b. Frontal lobe
c. Medulla
d. Thalamus
e. Pons

3-48. You are asked to evaluate Bob with the neurologist. The nurse in the office asks if you would like to order a CT (computed tomography) scan, and you request one. The CT scan shows that all the ventricles are dilated, especially the frontal horns of the lateral ventricles, without any evidence of obstruction by a tumor. What would be a possible mechanism underlying the enlargement of the ventricles?

a. Decreased CSF absorption
b. Low blood pressure
c. Decreased CNS blood flow
d. Decreased intracranial pressure
e. High blood pressure

3-49. If there is diminished CSF absorption, where does the blockage occur?

a. Pyramidal cells
b. Renshaw cells
c. Arachnoid villi
d. Purkinje cells
e. Sagittal sinus

3-50. Where would the greatest damage be done by the expanding ventricles?

a. Thalamus
b. Brainstem
c. Pituitary gland
d. Parietal cortex
e. Deep frontal white matter (corona radiata)

BLOCK 4

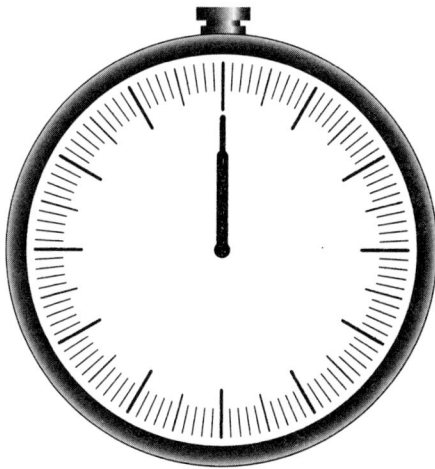

**YOU HAVE 60 MINUTES
TO COMPLETE 50 QUESTIONS.**

BLOCK 4

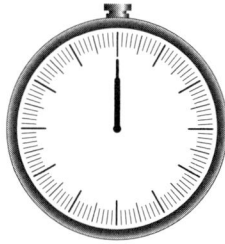

YOU HAVE *60* MINUTES
TO COMPLETE *50* QUESTIONS.

Questions

4-1. A 28-year-old male with AIDS returned from Haiti with acute diarrhea. The stool revealed an oval organism (8 to 9 micrometers in diameter) that was acid-fast and fluoresced blue under ultraviolet light. The most likely identification of this organism is

    a.   Cyclospora
    b.   Giardia
    c.   Enterocytozoon
    d.   Cryptosporidium
    e.   Prototheca

4-2. A 39-year-old male with gastroenteritis and no drug allergies is given an IV dose of antibiotic at a fast rate. As the antibiotic is infusing, the patient becomes flushed over most of his body. What antibiotic was given?

    a.   Vancomycin
    b.   Gentamicin
    c.   Erythromycin
    d.   Penicillin G
    e.   Tetracycline

4-3. A 35-year-old male presents with the new onset of a "bulge" in his left inguinal area. After performing your physical examination, you diagnose the "bulge" to be an inguinal hernia. You refer the patient to a surgeon who repairs the hernia and sends the resected hernia sac to the pathology laboratory along with some adipose tissue, which he calls a "lipoma of the cord." The pathology resident examines the tissue grossly, microscopically, and decides that it is not a neoplastic lipoma, but instead is non-neoplastic normal adipose tissue. Which one of the following features would have been present had the lesion been a lipoma rather than normal adipose tissue?

a. Anaplasia
b. Fibrous capsule
c. Numerous mitoses
d. Prominent nucleoli
e. Uniform population of cells

4-4. A 64-year-old male presents with recurrent chest pain that develops whenever he attempts to mow the grass in his yard. He relates that the pain goes away after a couple of minutes if he stops and rests. He also states that the pain has not increased in frequency or duration in the last several months. What is the most likely diagnosis for this patient?

a. Stable angina
b. Unstable angina
c. Atypical angina
d. Prinzmetal angina
e. Myocardial infarction

4-5. A 7-year-old boy accidentally inhales a small peanut (he was trying to see if it would fit inside his nose), and the peanut lodges in one of his bronchi. A chest x-ray reveals the mediastinum to be shifted toward the side of the obstruction. The best description for the lung changes that result from this obstruction is

a. Absorptive atelectasis
b. Compression atelectasis
c. Contraction atelectasis
d. Patchy atelectasis
e. Hyaline membrane disease

4-6. A 29-year-old female presents with severe pain during menstruation (dysmenorrhea). During work-up an endometrial biopsy is obtained. The pathology report from this specimen makes the diagnosis of chronic endometritis. Based on this pathology report, which one of the following was present in the biopsy sample of the endometrium?

a. Neutrophils
b. Lymphocytes
c. Lymphoid follicles
d. Plasma cells
e. Decidualized stromal cells

4-7. Damage to which structure in particular causes Sam's problem with movement?

a. Substantia gelatinosa
b. Substantia nigra, pars reticularis
c. Substantia nigra, pars compacta
d. Caudate nucleus
e. Thalamus

4-8. What is the blood supply of the main structure damaged?

a. Lenticulostriate branches of the middle cerebral and anterior cerebral arteries
b. Perforating branches of the basilar and vertebral arteries
c. Anterior choroidal artery and anterior cerebral artery
d. Posteromedial branches of the posterior cerebral and posterior communicating arteries
e. Anterior cerebral and anterior communicating arteries

4-9. What neurotransmitter is deficient?

a. Norepinephrine
b. Glutamate
c. Dopamine
d. Acetylcholine
e. GABA

4-10. Which of the following is a precursor to the deficient neurotransmitter and can be given as a medication to improve Sam's movement?

a. Tyrosine
b. Choline
c. Acetyl-CoA
d. Tryptamine
e. L-dopa

4-11. A 48-year-old female with a history of pituitary surgery and irradiation is scheduled for elective surgery. She currently requires replacement thyroxine, hydrocortisone, estrogen, and progesterone. In the perioperative period, you will treat her with

a. Glucose infusion
b. Increased hydrocortisone
c. ACTH infusion
d. Increased estrogen
e. Increased thyroxine

4-12. A 34-year-old mental patient frequently shouts in the halls of his psychiatric ward, disrupting activities and annoying the other patients. The best behavioral strategy for this patient would be

a. Psychological counseling
b. Contingency management
c. Stimulus control
d. Role-play therapy
e. Modeling

4-13. A 49-year-old male who smokes two packs of cigarettes a day presents with a lung mass on x-ray and recent weight gain. Laboratory examination shows hyponatremia with hyperosmolar urine. The patient probably has

a. Renal failure
b. Pituitary failure
c. Conn's syndrome
d. Cardiac failure
e. Inappropriate ADH

4-14. A 28-year-old male young skier with normal pulmonary function (minute volume 4L; pulmonary blood flow 5 L/ min) who is recovering from a tibial fracture suddenly develops right-sided chest pain and tachypnea. Embolic occlusion of the right pulmonary artery is suspected. The diagnosis would be immediately confirmed by which of the following alveolar gas measurements?

	P_{O_2} (mmHg)	P_{CO_2} (mmHg)
a.	125	60
b.	125	20
c.	100	40
d.	80	20
e.	80	60

4-15. An 35-year-old male presents with the sudden onset of massive diarrhea. Grossly, this individual's stool has the appearance of "rice-water" because of the presence of flecks of mucus. Cultures of this patient's stool grow *Vibrio cholera*, a curved, gram-negative rod that secretes an enterotoxin consisting of a toxic A subunit and a binding B subunit. The cholera enterotoxin causes massive diarrhea by

a. Inhibiting the conversion of Gi-GDP to Gi-GTP
b. Inhibiting the conversion of Gs-GTP to Gs-GDP
c. Stimulating the conversion of Gi-GDP to Gi-GTP
d. Stimulating the conversion of Gs-GDP to Gs-GTP
e. Stimulating the conversion of Gs-GTP to Gs-GDP

4-16. A 3-month-old male infant is being evaluated for severe neurological defects involving both of his legs, his urinary bladder, and his rectum. Physical examination reveals a cystic structure in his sacrolumbar region. Further examination reveals that this cystic structure contains meninges and portions of the spinal cord. What is the best diagnosis?

a. Anencephaly
b. Infantile hemiplegia
c. Myeloschisis
d. Spina bifida with meningocele
e. Spina bifida with meningomyelocele

4-17. A 51-year-old male alcoholic with a history of chronic liver disease presents with increasing weight loss and ascites. Physical examination reveals a slightly enlarged, soft, nontender prostate. Examination of the scrotum is unremarkable, and fecal occult blood tests are negative. A chest x-ray is unremarkable, but a CT scan of the abdomen reveals a single mass in the left lobe of the liver. Work-up reveals elevated levels of α-fetoprotein in this patient's blood. At this point the most likely diagnosis for the liver mass is

a. Angiosarcoma
b. Cholangiocarcinoma
c. Hepatoblastoma
d. Hepatocellular carcinoma
e. Metastatic colon cancer

4-18. A 38-year-old male presents with multiple café-au-lait spots and neurofibromas. His father and mother do not have neurofibromas. This may be an example of

a. A new mutation
b. Hypermorphism
c. A dominant negative mutation
d. Antimorphism

4-19. A 22-year-old male comes to the emergency room of your hospital because he has a diffuse, erythematous rash involving nearly all of his body. His total WBC count is greater than 100,000 cells/mm^3. He also complains of bone pain, severe irritability, weakness, fatigue, nausea and vomiting, constipation, photophobia, and polyuria. His electrocardiogram (ECG) shows shortening of the QT interval, prolongation of the PR interval, and nonspecific T-wave changes. The most likely cause of his symptoms is

a. Hypercalcemia
b. Hypocalcemia
c. Hypophosphatemia
d. Hyperkalemia

4-20. A young female of average intelligence and short stature who has never menstruated is under clinical investigation for Turner's syndrome. However, a buccal smear shows some cells with one Barr body. Which of the following best explains this finding?

a. Laboratory error
b. The patient is a male
c. Classic XO pattern
d. Turner's mosaic pattern
e. Klinefelter's syndrome

4-21. A nine-year-old male is diagnosed with acute lymphoblastic leukemia. He is maintained on methotrexate. A recent platelet count is below normal, and a stool guaiac is 4+. Which of the following agents should be administered to counteract methotrexate toxicity?

a. N-acetylcysteine
b. Vitamin K
c. Penicillamine
d. Leucovorin
e. Deferoxamine

4-22. A physician examines a 36-year-old patient who complains of pain and paresthesia in the left leg. The distribution of the pain—running down the medial aspect of the leg and the medial side of the foot and including the great toe—is suggestive of a herniated intervertebral disk. The physician links the distribution of symptoms with nerve L4 and concludes that herniation has occurred at which location?

a. L3–L4 intervertebral disk
b. L4–L5 intervertebral disk
c. L5–S1 intervertebral disk
d. S1–S2 intervertebral disk
e. Insufficient data to determine

4-23. A 30-year-old female presents with a 6-month history of amenorrhea. Your initial evaluation should include measurement of

a. Prolactin
b. Estradiol
c. Progesterone
d. Testosterone
e. DHEA-S

4-24. A 35-year-old male has a prolactinoma and a history of severe peptic ulcer disease. There is a family history of pituitary tumors. The findings of what other diagnostic test at this time may be abnormal and potentially useful in diagnosis?

a. Fasting blood sugar
b. Serum calcium
c. Serum calcitonin
d. Urinary metanephrine
e. Serum ferritin

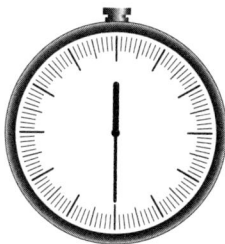

YOU SHOULD HAVE COMPLETED APPROXIMATELY *25 QUESTIONS AND HAVE* *30 MINUTES REMAINING.*

Clinical Case (Questions 4-25 through 4-28)

A second-year medical student was asked to see a nursing home patient as a requirement for a Physical Diagnosis course. The patient was a 79-year-old male who was apparently in a coma. The student wasn't certain of how to approach this case, so he asked the patient's wife, who was sitting at the bedside, why this patient was in a coma. The wife replied: "Oh, Paul isn't in a coma. But he did have a stroke." Slightly confused, the student leaned over and asked Paul to open his eyes. He opened his eyes immediately. However, when asked to lift his arm or speak, Paul did nothing. The student than asked Paul's wife if she was certain that his eye opening was not simply a coincidence, and that he really was in a coma, since he was unable to follow any commands.

Paul's wife explained that he was unable to move or speak as a result of his stroke. However, she knew that he was awake, because he could communicate with her by blinking his eyes. The student appeared rather skeptical, so Paul's wife asked her husband to blink once for "yes" and twice for "no." She then asked him if he was at home and he blinked twice. When asked if he were in a nursing home, he blinked once. The student than asked him to move his eyes, and he was able to look in his direction. However, when the student asked him if he could move his arms or legs, he blinked twice. He also blinked twice when asked if he could smile. He did the same when asked if he could feel someone moving his arm. The student thanked Paul and his wife for their time, made notes of his findings, and returned to class.

4-25. Where in the nervous system could a lesion occur that can cause paralysis of the extremities bilaterally, as well as the face, but not of the eyes?

a. High cervical spinal cord bilaterally
b. Bilateral thalamus
c. Bilateral basal ganglia
d. Bilateral pontine tegmentum
e. Bilateral frontal lobe

4-26. An infarct in what vascular distribution could cause this lesion?

a. Anterior spinal artery
b. Vertebral artery
c. Basilar artery
d. Middle cerebral artery
e. Posterior cerebral artery

4-27. Damage to which tracts caused Paul's inability to move his arms and legs?

a. Corticospinal and corticobulbar tracts
b. Spinothalamic tract
c. Tractus solitarius
d. Brachium conjunctivum
e. Superior cerebellar peduncle

4-28. Damage to which tract caused Paul's lack of perception of someone moving his arm?

a. Corticospinal and corticobulbar
b. Middle cerebellar peduncle
c. Spinothalamic tract
d. Rubrospinal tract
e. Medial lemniscus

4-29. A patient with a malabsorption syndrome who develops a deficiency of vitamin A is most likely to develop which one of the following abnormalities?

a. Acute leukemia
b. Intestinal metaplasia
c. Megaloblastic anemia
d. Night blindness
e. Soft bones

4-30. A 30-year-old male presents with multiple soft, raised, beefy-red superficial ulcers in his left groin. Physical examination reveals several enlarged left inguinal lymph nodes. A histologic section from an enlarged lymph node that is stained with a silver stain reveals characteristic "Donovan bodies" within macrophages. What is the most likely diagnosis?

a. Chancroid
b. Gonorrhea
c. Granuloma inguinale
d. Lymphogranuloma venereum
e. Syphilis

4-31. A 34-year-old male presents with the sudden development of malaise along with dyspnea, fever, and a cough. You discover that approximately 5 hours prior to developing these symptoms he had been working with moldy hay, and this exposure led to the production of his symptoms. What is your diagnosis?

a. Farmer's lung
b. Bagassosis
c. Byssinosis
d. Progressive massive fibrosis
e. Pigeon breeder's disease

4-32. An infant, seen in ER, presented with a fever and persistent cough. Physical examination and a chest x-ray suggested pneumonia. Which of the following is most likely the cause of this infection?

a. Rotavirus
b. Adenovirus
c. Coxsackievirus
d. Respiratory syncytial virus
e. Rhinovirus

4-33. A 26-year-old female comatose laboratory technician is rushed into the emergency room. She dies while you are examining her. Her most dramatic symptom is that her body is literally hot to your touch, indicating an extremely high fever. You learn that her lab has been working on metabolic inhibitors and that there is a high likelihood that she accidentally ingested one. Which one of the following is the most likely culprit?

a. Barbiturates
b. Piericidin A
c. Dimercaprol
d. Dinitrophenol
e. Cyanide

4-34. A 29-year-old male uses secobarbital to satisfy his addiction to barbiturates. During the past week, he is imprisoned and is not able to obtain the drug. He is brought to the prison medical ward because of the onset of severe anxiety, increased sensitivity to light, dizziness, and generalized tremors. On physical examination, he is hyperreflexic. Which of the following agents should he be given to diminish his withdrawal symptoms?

a. Buspirone
b. Chloral hydrate
c. Chlorpromazine
d. Diazepam
e. Trazodone

4-35. A 37-year-old female presents with a lump in the upper outer quadrant of the left breast, which shows a wide spectrum of benign breast disease on pathologic examination. Which of the following is considered to indicate the greatest risk for subsequent carcinoma of the breast?

a. Intraductal papillomatosis
b. Sclerosing adenosis
c. Focal papillomatosis
d. Marked apocrine metaplasia
e. Epithelial hyperplasia of the ducts

4-36. A 32-year-old female sees her physician because of "stiffness" and intolerance to cold temperatures in her fingers. Her face has a "masklike" quality. It would be appropriate in the systems review to ask about

a. Headaches and dizziness
b. Swallowing difficulties
c. Sun hypersensitivity
d. Thyroid trouble
e. Family history

4-37. A 48-year-old male taking an oral sulfonamide is found to have a markedly decreased peripheral blood neutrophil count, but the number of platelets and erythrocytes are normal. If the peripheral neutropenia is the result of antineutrophile antibodies being produced in response to taking the sulfonamide, then this patient would be expected to have

a. An atrophic spleen
b. Decreased vitamin B12 levels
c. Hypoplasia of the bone marrow myeloid series
d. Hyperplasia of the bone marrow myeloid series
e. A monoclonal large granular lymphocyte proliferation in the peripheral blood

4-38. A 24-year-old female delivers a normal 8-pound baby boy at 40 weeks of gestation. She has no history of drug abuse, and her pregnancy was unremarkable. Examination had revealed the placenta to be located normally, but following delivery she fails to deliver the placenta and subsequently develops massive postpartum hemorrhage and shock. Emergency surgery is performed to stop the bleeding. Her postpartum bleeding was most likely caused by

a. An abruptio placenta
b. A placenta previa
c. A placenta accreta
d. A hydatidiform mole
e. An invasive mole

4-39. A 28-year-old female believes that she might be infertile. She had a healthy child 3 years ago and has been trying to get pregnant with the child's father for the last 18 months. There is no dysmenorrhea. Her menses occur regularly but have significantly less flow as compared with prior to the pregnancy. She recalls having a curettage performed to remove placental remnants. What is the diagnosis?

a. Ovarian failure
b. Hypothyroidism
c. Asherman's syndrome
d. Endometriosis
e. Prolactinoma

4-40. A teenage baseball player was hit in the base of the skull by a loose bat. The patient is hoarse and complains of difficulty swallowing. The cranial x-ray indicates a basal skull fracture which passes through the jugular foramen.

The examining physician notes a large hematoma behind the ear on the injured side. This is most likely the result of damage to

a. A branch of the internal carotid artery
b. The external jugular vein
c. The occipital artery
d. The posterior auricular artery
e. The superficial temporal artery

Clinical Case (Questions 4-41 through 4-44)

Joe is a 75-year-old male who is right-handed and was told in the past by his internist that he had an irregular heartbeat. Unfortunately, Joe decided that he didn't wish to learn anything further about this condition, so he didn't return to this physician and it remained untreated. One morning, he awoke to find that his face drooped on the right side, and that he couldn't move his right arm or right leg. When he tried to call an ambulance for help, he had a great deal of difficulty communicating with the operator because his speech was slurred, non-fluent, and missing some pronouns. The call was traced by the police, and an ambulance arrived at his house and brought him to an emergency room.

A neurologist was called to see Joe in the emergency room. When he listened to Joe's heart, he detected an irregular heartbeat. It was very difficult to understand Joe's speech, because it was halting, with a tendency to repeat the same phrases over and over. He had a great deal of difficulty repeating specific sentences given to him by the neurologist, but he was able to follow simple commands such as: "touch your right ear with your left hand." His mouth drooped on the right when he attempted to smile, but his forehead remained symmetric when he wrinkled it. He couldn't move his right arm at all, but was able to wiggle his right leg a little bit.

4-41. What kind of language problem does Joe have?

a. Dysarthria
b. Wernicke's aphasia
c. Broca's aphasia
d. Alexia
e. Pure word deafness

4-42. Which area of the brain is damaged?

a. Internal capsule and thalamus
b. Right occipital lobe
c. Pontine reticular formation
d. Corpus callosum
e. Left pre-central gyrus and Broca's area

4-43. Which artery was blocked when the event occurred?

a. Anterior cerebral artery
b. Posterior cerebral artery
c. Anterior inferior cerebellar artery
d. Middle cerebral artery
e. Basilar artery

4-44. Which term best describes Joe's facial weakness?

a. Peripheral VII nerve
b. Central VII nerve
c. XII nerve
d. V nerve
e. Oculomotor nerve weakness

4-45. A 29-year-old female has had three spontaneous (unplanned) abortions. All three occurred at approximately 6 weeks gestational age. The results of her physical exam are normal. Which of these may be the cause?

a. Ovary
b. Thyroid gland
c. Adrenal gland
d. Pituitary gland

4-46. A 34-year-old male patient visited a physician with complaints of fatigue, weight loss, night sweats, and "swollen glands." The physician also observed that he had an oral yeast infection. Which of the following tests would most likely reveal the cause of his problems?

a. A test for CD8 lymphocytes
b. An HTLV I test
c. An HIV ELISA test
d. A test for infectious mononucleosis
e. A test for *Candida albicans*

4-47. A patient who presents to the hospital with severe headaches developed convulsions and died. At autopsy the brain grossly had a "Swiss cheese" appearance due to the presence of numerous small cysts containing milky fluid. Microscopically, a scolex with hooklets is found within one of these cysts. What is the causative agent for this disease?

a. *Taenia saginata*
b. *Taenia solium*
c. *Diphyllobothrium latum*
d. *Echinococcus granulosa*
e. *Toxocara canis*

4-48. A 37-year-old female who has a clinical picture of fever, splenomegaly, varying neurologic manifestations, and purplish ecchymoses of the skin is found to have a hemoglobin level of 10.0 g/dL, a mean corpuscular hemoglobin concentration (MCHC) of 48, peripheral blood polychromasia with stippled macrocytes, and spherocytes, with a blood urea nitrogen level of 68 mg/dL. The findings of coagulation studies and the patient's fibrin-degraded products are not overtly abnormal. Which of the following is most closely identified with these findings?

a. Idiopathic thrombocytopenic purpura
b. Thrombotic thrombocytopenic purpura
c. Disseminated intravascular coagulopathy
d. Submassive hepatic necrosis
e. Waterhouse-Friderichsen syndrome

4-49. A 10-month old, previously healthy, male infant develops a severe, watery diarrhea 2 days after visiting the pediatrician for a routine checkup. The most likely diagnosis is

a. Rotavirus infection
b. Enterotoxigenic *E. coli* infection
c. *Entamoeba histolytica* infection
d. Lactase deficiency
e. Ulcerative colitis

4-50. At a follow-up visit one month after a 22-year-old male was newly diagnosed with schizophrenia and started on chlorpromazine, he has several complaints, listed below. Which of them CANNOT be attributed to chlorpromazine?

a. A "restless feeling"
b. Sexual dysfunction
c. Urinary hesitancy
d. Vomiting

BLOCK 5

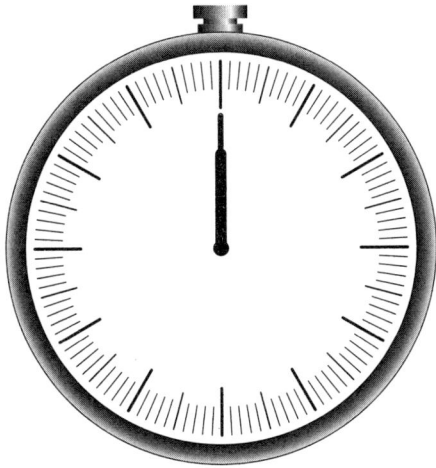

**YOU HAVE 60 MINUTES
TO COMPLETE 50 QUESTIONS.**

BLOCK 5

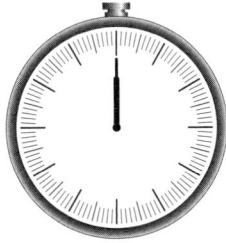

You have **60** *minutes*
to complete **50** *questions.*

Questions

Clinical Case (Questions 5-1 through 5-4)

Gary is a 35-year-old male who was previously healthy until one day he noticed that his right leg was weak. As the day progressed, he found that he was dragging the leg behind him when he walked, and he finally asked a friend to drive him home from work because he was unable to lift his right foot up enough to place it on the gas pedal. He also noticed that his left leg felt a little bit numb. Finally, his wife convinced him to go to the emergency room of his local hospital.

When Gary arrived at the emergency room, he was having a great deal of difficulty walking. The physician who examined him asked him when this began, and when Gary thought about it in more depth, he realized that perhaps this had started slowly several days before, and he had ignored the symptoms. Gary's language function, cranial nerves, and motor and sensory examinations of his arms were within normal limits. When the physician examined Gary's right leg, it was markedly weak, with very brisk reflexes in the knee and ankle. Vibration and position sense in the right leg were absent. Pain and temperature testing were normal in the right leg, but these sensations were absent on the left leg and abdomen to the level of his

75

umbilicus. Reflexes in the left leg were normal, but when the physician scratched the lateral portion of the plantar surface on the bottom side of Gary's right foot, the big toe moved up. The remainder of Gary's examination was normal.

5-1. What area of the nervous system is damaged?

a. Brainstem
b. Cervical spinal cord
c. Thoracic spinal cord
d. Frontal lobe
e. Peripheral nerves

5-2. Damage to which tract could give Gary the loss of vibration and position sense on the right side?

a. Right fasciculus cuneatus
b. Right fasciculus gracilis
c. Left fasciculus cuneatus
d. Left fasciculus gracilis
e. Right Lissauer's tract

5-3. Gary's loss of left-sided pain and temperature sensation could be due to damage of which tract?

a. Right fasciculus cuneatus
b. Right fasciculus gracilis
c. Right spinothalamic tract
d. Left spinothalamic tract
e. Left corticospinal tract

5-4. Why is Gary's right leg weak?

a. There is muscle damage in the right leg
b. There is damage in his left frontal lobe
c. There is damage to the right corticospinal tract
d. The dorsal root is damaged
e. There is damage to the right femoral nerve

5-5. A 13-year-old child with blue scleras, mildly short stature, no deformity, and a past history significant for 10 fractured bones most likely has

a. Type I osteogenesis imperfecta
b. Type II osteogenesis imperfecta
c. Type III osteogenesis imperfecta
d. Type IV osteogenesis imperfecta

5-6. A 42-year-old male presents because recently he has had to change his shoe size from 9 to 10½. He also says that his hands and jaw are now larger. The disorder is most likely mediated through the actions of excess

a. Prolactin
b. ACTH
c. Somatomedin
d. Antidiuretic hormone
e. Thyrotropin

5-7. A 24-year-old male presents with a large wound to his right forearm that is the result of a chain-saw accident. You treat his wound appropriately and follow him in your surgery clinic at routine intervals. Initially his wound is filled with granulation tissue, which is composed of proliferating fibroblasts and proliferating new blood vessels (*angiogenesis*). A growth factor that is capable of inducing all the steps necessary for angiogenesis is

a.   Epidermal growth factor (EGF)
b.   Transforming growth factor α (TGF-α)
c.   Platelet-derived growth factor (PDGF)
d.   Basic fibroblast growth factor (FGF)
e.   Transforming growth factor β (TGF-β)

5-8. A 45-year-old male during a routine physical examination is found to have microscopic hematuria. Further work-up finds a 4.5 cm mass in the upper pole of his right kidney. This mass is resected and reveals a tumor composed of a uniform population of cells with clear cytoplasm. Mitoses are not found. Further work-up fails to reveal the presence of any metastatic disease. Based on all of these findings, which of the following best characterizes this tumor? (Note: Assume that a low stage has a better prognosis than a high stage, and a low grade has a better prognosis than a high grade. Also assume that renal tumors composed of cells with clear cytoplasm that are larger than 2.0 cm in diameter are malignant.)

Tumor	Grade	Stage
a. Benign	Not applicable	Not applicable
b. Malignant	Low	Low
c. Malignant	Low	High
d. Malignant	High	Low
e. Malignant	High	High

5-9. A 35-year-old female who lives in the southeastern portion of the United States and likes to hike in the Great Smoky Mountains presents with a spotted rash that started on her extremities and spread to her trunk and face. A biopsy of one of these lesions revealed necrosis and reactive hyperplasia of blood vessels. What is the most likely causative agent of her disease?

a. *Bartonella henselae*
b. *Bartonella quintana*
c. *Coxiella burnetii*
d. *Rickettsia prowazekii*
e. *Rickettsia rickettsii*

5-10. A 39-year-old female presents with increasing shortness of breath. She states that for the past 6 months she has been taking an unauthorized appetite suppressant to try to lose weight. Physical examination reveals signs of right heart failure. She is admitted to the hospital to work-up her symptoms, but she dies suddenly. A section from her heart at the time of autopsy reveals marked thickening of the right ventricle, but the thickness of the left ventricle is within normal limits. The endocardium does not appear to be increased in thickness or fibrotic, and the cardiac valves do not appear abnormal. Neither ventricular cavity is dilated. Which one of the following best describes this cardiac pathology?

a. Carcinoid heart disease
b. Cor pulmonale
c. Eccentric hypertrophy
d. Systemic hypertensive heart disease
e. Volume overload to the heart

5-11. A firefighter, age 34 and a nonsmoker, complains of bouts of dizziness at times of intense exertion. His history reveals having been exposed to intense smoke 6 months ago when his breathing apparatus malfunctioned during a job. He is scheduled for a pulmonary function test.

The patient is connected to the spirometer. He is asked to relax and breathe normally to establish a baseline. The pump-handle movement (elevation of the manubrium) during inspiration involves all the following EXCEPT

a. Increase in the anterior-posterior chest diameter
b. Increase in the superior-inferior chest diameter
c. Movement at the costovertebral joints
d. Movement at the sternomandibular joint

5-12. A 75-year-old female in CHF is unable to climb a flight of stairs without experiencing shortness of breath. Digoxin is administered to improve cardiac muscle contractility. Within two weeks, she has a marked improvement in her symptoms. What cellular action of digoxin accounts for this?

a. Inhibition of cyclic adenosine monophosphate (AMP) synthesis
b. Inhibition of mitochondrial Ca release
c. Inhibition of the sodium (Na) pump
d. Inhibition of β-adrenergic stimulation
e. Inhibition of adenosine triphosphate (ATP) degradation

5-13. An 8-month-old infant presents with progressive renal and hepatic failure. Despite intensive medical therapy, this young infant dies. At the time of autopsy the external surface of his kidneys were found to be smooth, but the cut section revealed numerous cysts that were lined up in a row. What is the mode of inheritance of this renal abnormality?

a. Autosomal dominant
b. Autosomal recessive
c. X-linked dominant
d. X-linked recessive
e. Mitochondrial

5-14. A 27-year-old female in the last trimester of her first pregnancy presents with the sudden onset of multiple skin hemorrhages. She states that for the past several days she has not felt the baby move. Work-up reveals an increase in the PT and PTT, while fibrin degradation products (FDP) are increased in her blood. Her platelet count is found to be 43,000/µL. What is the most likely diagnosis for this patient?

a. Autoimmune thrombocytopenia purpura (autoimmune ITP)
b. Isoimmune thrombocytopenia purpura (isoimmune ITP)
c. Thrombotic thrombocytopenia purpura (TTP)
d. Hemolytic uremic syndrome (HUS)
e. Disseminated intravascular coagulation (DIC)

5-15. A 3 cm mass is found in the right upper lobe (RUL) of a 48-year-old male long-term smoker during a routine physical examination. Histologic examination of a trans-bronchial biopsy specimen reveals infiltrating groups of cells with scant cytoplasm. No glandular structures or keratin production are seen. The nuclei of these cells are small, round, and do not appear to have nucleoli. Electron microscopy reveals membrane-bound dense core neurosecretory granules. What is your diagnosis?

a. Adenocarcinoma
b. Hamartoma
c. Large cell undifferentiated carcinoma
d. Small cell carcinoma
e. Squamous cell carcinoma

5-16. A 28-year-old previously healthy female, with no past medical history, is now 28 weeks pregnant. She complains of trouble seeing, polyuria, polyphagia, and polydipsia. What is her diagnosis?

a. Gestational diabetes mellitus
b. Deep venous thrombosis
c. Urinary tract infection
d. Preeclampsia

5-17. A 68-year-old male with a peptic ulcer was admitted to the hospital and a gastric biopsy was performed. The tissue was cultured on chocolate agar incubated in a microaerophilic environment at 37°C for 5 to 7 days. At 5 days of incubation, colonies appeared on the plate and were curved, gram-negative rods, oxidase-positive. The most likely identity of this organism is

a. *Campylobacter jejuni*
b. *Vibrio parahaemolyticus*
c. *Haemophilus influenzae*
d. *Helicobacter* (previously *Campylobacter*) *pylori*
e. *Campylobacter fetus*

5-18. A 28-year-old female develops galactorrhea without amenorrhea. Your evaluation should include

a. Estradiol
b. Progesterone
c. Prolactin
d. Testosterone
e. DHEA-S

5-19. A 19-year-old female has galactorrhea. She has never been pregnant. Which hormone is the most likely to be responsible for this situation?

a. Prolactin
b. Estrogen
c. Progesterone
d. Thyroxine
e. Cortisol

5-20. A 54-year-old male presents with a high fever, jaundice, and colicky abdominal pain in the right upper quadrant. The gallbladder cannot be palpated by physical examination. Work-up reveals hemoglobin level of 15.3 g/dL, unconjugated bilirubin level of 0.9 mg/dL, conjugated bilirubin level of 1.1 mg/dL, and alkaline phosphatase level of 180 IU/L. What is the best diagnosis?

a. Acute cholecystitis
b. Chronic cholecystitis
c. Bile duct obstruction by a stone
d. Carcinoma of the gallbladder
e. Carcinoma of the head of the pancreas

5-21. A 25-year-old female presents to your office for work-up of infertility. In taking a history she describes severe pain during menses, and she also tells you that in the past another doctor told her that she had "chocolate in her cysts." Based on this history, what abnormality would you most expect to be present in this patient?

a. Metastatic ovarian cancer
b. Endometriosis
c. Acute pelvic inflammatory disease
d. Adenomyosis
e. A posteriorly located subserosal uterine leiomyoma

5-22. A 70-year-old female is brought to the emergency room by her granddaughter because she has developed ecchymosis covering many areas of her body. Her granddaughter states that her grandmother lives alone at home and has not been eating well. Her diet has consisted of mainly tea and toast, as she does not eat milk, fruits, or vegetables. Your physical examination reveals small hemorrhages around hair follicles, some of these follicles having an unusual "cork-screw" appearance. You also notice swelling and hemorrhages of her gingiva. What is the most likely diagnosis?

a. Beriberi
b. Kwashiorkor
c. Pellagra
d. Rickets
e. Scurvy

5-23. A 27-year-old male presents with reactive depression following the accidental death of a close relative. A tricyclic antidepressant is chosen to control his depression. Which adverse effects would NOT be of concern?

a. Disturbance in rapid-eye-movement (REM) sleep
b. Sedation
c. Dry mouth
d. Orthostatic hypotension
e. Tardive dyskinesia

5-24. A 62-year-old female is unable to hear high frequency sounds. The damage to the basilar membrane is closest to the

a. Oval window
b. Helicotrema
c. Stria vascularis
d. Modiolus
e. Spiral ganglion

5-25. A 15-year-old phenotypically female patient presents for workup of primary amenorrhea and is found to have an XY karyotype. The most likely diagnosis is

a. Turner's syndrome
b. Mixed gonadal dysgenesis
c. True hermaphroditism
d. Male pseudohermaphroditism
e. Female pseudohermaphroditism

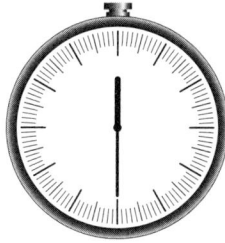

YOU SHOULD HAVE COMPLETED APPROXIMATELY
25 QUESTIONS AND HAVE 30 MINUTES REMAINING.

5-26. An 87-year-old male develops worsening heart failure. Work-up reveals decreased left ventricular filling due to decreased compliance of the left ventricle. Two months later this patient dies, and postmortem sections reveal deposits of eosinophilic, Congo red-positive material in the interstitium of his heart. When viewed under polarized light, this material displays an apple-green birefringence. What is your diagnosis?

a. Amyloidosis
b. Glycogenosis
c. Hemochromatosis
d. Sarcoidosis
e. Senile atrophy

5-27. In a program aimed at cessation of smoking, a 45-year-old female is required to smoke many cigarettes in a small booth and over a short period of time. Which technique can best help her?

a. Habituation
b. Aversive conditioning
c. Stimulus control
d. Variable-ratio reinforcement
e. Systematic desensitization

Clinical Case (Questions 5-28 through 5-31)

Emma is a 64-year-old female who has had heart disease for many years. While carrying chemicals down the stairs of the dry cleaning shop where she worked, she suddenly lost control of her right leg and arm. She fell down the stairs and was able to stand up with some assistance from a co-worker. When attempting to walk on her own, she had a very unsteady gait, with a tendency to fall to the right side. Her supervisor asked her if she was all right, and noticed that her speech was very slurred when she tried to answer. He called an ambulance to take her to the nearest hospital.

The physician who was called to see Emma in the emergency room noted that her speech was slurred as if she were intoxicated, but the grammar and meaning were intact. Her face appeared symmetric, but when asked to protrude her tongue, it deviated toward the left. She was unable to tell if her right toe was moved up or down by the physician when she closed her eyes, and couldn't feel the buzz of a tuning fork on her right arm and leg. In addition, her right arm and leg were markedly weak. The physician could find no other abnormalities on the remainder of Emma's general medical examination.

5-28. Where in the nervous system has the damage occurred?

a. Right lateral medulla
b. Occipital lobe
c. Left lateral medulla
d. Right cervical spinal cord
e. Left medial medulla

5-29. Where in the nervous system could a lesion occur that causes arm and leg weakness, but spares the face?

a. Right corticospinal tract in the cervical spinal cord
b. Left inferior frontal lobe
c. Left medullary pyramids
d. Occipital lobe
e. Both A and C

5-30. Other than the weakness on her right side, what type of deficit could cause Emma's gait problem and where could a lesion causing this deficit occur?

a. Proprioceptive, left medial lemniscus
b. Sight, left eye
c. Proprioceptive, descending component of the MLF
d. Pain, left spinothalamic tract
e. Proprioceptive, right medial lemniscus

5-31. Deviation of the tongue to the left, away from the right hemiparesis, implies a lesion in which area of the nervous system?

a. Right hypoglossal nucleus
b. Left hypoglossal nucleus
c. Right inferior frontal lobe
d. Left inferior frontal lobe
e. There is no lesion that causes this

5-32. A 68-year-old female presents with a single, uniformly brown round lesion that appears to be "stuck on" the right side of her face. Histologic sections from this lesion reveal hyperkeratosis with horn and pseudo-horn cyst formation. What is the correct diagnosis for this skin lesion?

a.   Seborrheic keratosis
b.   Squamous cell carcinoma
c.   Verruca vulgaris
d.   Keratoacanthoma
e.   Actinic keratosis

5-33. Two days after receiving the antimalarial drug primaquine, a 27-year-old black male developed sudden intravascular hemolysis resulting in a decreased hematocrit, hemoglobinemia, and hemoglobinuria. Examination of the peripheral blood revealed erythrocytes with a membrane defect forming "bite" cells; when crystal violet stain was applied, many Heinz bodies were seen. The most likely diagnosis is

a.   Hereditary spherocytosis
b.   Glucose-6-phosphate dehydrogenase deficiency
c.   Paroxysmal nocturnal hemoglobinuria
d.   Autoimmune hemolytic anemia
e.   Microangiopathic hemolytic anemia

5-34. A young female with lower pelvic pain, menometrorrhagia, and a negative β-hCG test undergoes uterine dilatation and curettage. The pathology report on the endometrial sample states, "Compatible with decidualized gestational hyperplasia, no chorionic villi present." The next step would be to

a.   Repeat the β-hCG test
b.   Discharge the patient
c.   Consider ectopic pregnancy
d.   Consider appendicitis
e.   Consider pelvic inflammatory disease

5-35. A 45-year-old white male with a limited small cell lung cancer presents to the emergency room of a local hospital and exhibits agitation and confusion, ataxia, nystagmus, peripheral sensory loss, and generalized weakness. The most likely etiology of this disorder is

a.   Hypercalcemia
b.   Paraneoplastic syndrome
c.   Cerebral vascular accident
d.   Myasthenia gravis

5-36. A 23-year-old female presents with weakness and amenorrhea. She is clinically hypothyroid. A CT scan of the pituitary shows an expanded sella with a large cystic component with calcifications. The most likely diagnosis is

a.   Pituitary macroadenoma
b.   Empty-sella syndrome
c.   Craniopharyngioma
d.   Optic glioma
e.   Hypothalamic hamartoma

5-37. A teenage female was brought to the Medical Center because of her complaints that she got too tired when asked to participate in gym class. A consulting neurologist found muscle weakness in her arms and legs. When no obvious diagnosis could be made, biopsies of her muscles were taken for tests. Chemistries revealed greatly elevated amounts of triacylglycerides esterified with primarily long chain fatty acids. Pathology reported the presence of significant numbers of lipid vacuoles in the muscle biopsy. Which one of the following is the most likely diagnosis?

a. Fatty acid synthase deficiency
b. Tay-Sachs disease
c. Carnitine deficiency
d. Biotin deficiency
e. Lipoprotein lipase deficiency

5-38. A 75-year-old female is hospitalized for pneumonia and treated with an IV antibiotic. On day three, she develops severe diarrhea. Stool is positive for *Clostridium difficile* toxin. What is the best treatment?

a. Clindamycin
b. Cefaclor
c. Vancomycin
d. Erythromycin

5-39. During a viral infection, a 23-year-old female develops enlarged lymph nodes at multiple sites (lymphadenopathy). A biopsy from one of these enlarged lymph nodes reveals a proliferative of reactive T immunoblasts, cells that have prominent nucleoli. These reactive T cells are most likely to be found in which one of the following regions of the lymph node?

a. Hilum
b. Medullary sinuses
c. Paracortex
d. Primary follicles
e. Secondary follicles

5-40. A 5-year-old male presents with clumsiness, a waddling gait, and difficulty climbing steps. Physical examination reveals that he uses his arms and shoulder muscles to rise from the floor or the chair. Additionally, his calves appear to be somewhat larger than normal. The physical findings are most consistent with a diagnosis of

a. Inclusion body myositis
b. Werdnig-Hoffman disease
c. Dermatomyositis
d. Duchenne's muscular dystrophy
e. Myotonic dystrophy

Clinical Case (Questions 5-41 through 5-44)

Susan is a 32-year-old female who recently stopped taking her birth control pills in order to become pregnant. However, after several months, her menstrual period failed to resume. Prior to beginning the birth control pills several years before, she had been having normal cycles. She also noticed headaches, which had been increasing in severity over the past several months. Recently, she became aware of difficulty with her peripheral vision. Thinking that she might be pregnant, she sought the attention of her gynecologist.

Her doctor ran a pregnancy test, which was negative. She told her that there may be another cause of the absence of her menstrual cycle, and she sent Susan's blood for levels of various hormones. When Susan returned to find out the results of the tests, her gynecologist told her that the level of the hormone prolactin was high. Susan remembered her headaches and visual symptoms, and informed her doctor, who promptly referred her to a neurologist.

The neurologist listened to Susan's story, and examined her. She found only that Susan was unable to see fingers in the temporal fields (lateral half of each visual field) of both of her eyes. The remainder of her neurologic exam was normal. The neurologist told Susan that she would like to order an MRI (magnetic resonance imaging) test of her head, in order to find out why she had the headaches, visual problem, and high prolactin levels.

5-41. A tumor in which area could cause a high prolactin level?

a. Adenohypophysis
b. Neurohypophysis
c. Amygdala
d. Hippocampus
e. Adrenal gland

5-42. What type of neurologic visual loss can cause a loss of peripheral vision?

a. Central scotoma
b. Superior quadrantanopsia
c. Bitemporal hemianopsia
d. Homonymous hemianopsia
e. Papilledema

5-43. A lesion adjacent to which structure caused Susan's visual problem?

a. Optic nerve
b. Optic radiations
c. Retina
d. Optic chiasm
e. Lateral geniculate nucleus

5-44. Which hypothalamic nucleus regulates prolactin secretion?

a. Suprachiasmatic nucleus
b. Preoptic nucleus
c. Paraventricular nucleus
d. Supraoptic nucleus
e. Arcuate nucleus

5-45. A 32-year-old female medical technologist visited Scandinavia and consumed raw fish daily for 2 weeks. Six months after her return home, she had a routine physical and was found to be anemic. Her vitamin B12 levels were below normal. The most likely cause of her vitamin B12 deficiency anemia is

a. Excessive consumption of ice-cold vodka
b. Infection with parvovirus B19
c. Infection with the fish tapeworm *Diphyllobothrium latum*
d. Infection with Yersinia
e. Cysticercosis

5-46. A 45-year-old male has decreased libido and decreased sexual function. A large pituitary tumor is found. His prolactin is 20 (<15). Testing of his pituitary–gonadal axis most likely will demonstrate

a. Normal testosterone and low LH
b. High testosterone and normal LH
c. Low testosterone and low LH
d. Normal testosterone and normal LH
e. Low testosterone and high LH

5-47. A 47-year-old male dies suddenly five days following major surgery. At autopsy a large blood clot is found obstructing the bifurcation of the pulmonary arteries. No gross abnormalities are found within the heart. The pulmonary blood clot most likely originated in the

a. Femoral artery
b. Popliteal artery
c. Superficial leg veins
d. Deep leg veins
e. Tricuspid valve

5-48. An 18-year-old female presents with abdominal pain localized to the right lower quadrant, nausea and vomiting, mild fever, and an elevation of the peripheral leukocyte count to 17,000 cells per microliter. Examination of the surgically resected appendix is most likely to reveal

a. An appendix with normal appearance
b. Neutrophils within the muscular wall
c. Lymphoid hyperplasia and multinucleated giant cells within the muscular wall
d. A dilated lumen filled with mucus
e. A yellow tumor nodule at the tip of the appendix

5-49. A 72-year-old female with a long history of anxiety treated with diazepam decides to triple her dose because of increasing fearfulness about "environmental noises." Several days after her attempt at self-prescribing, her neighbor finds her to be extremely lethargic and non-responsive. On examination, she is found to be stuporous and have diminished reaction to pain and decreased reflexes. Her respiratory rate is 8 breaths per minute (BPM), and she has shallow respirations. Which antidote could be given to reverse these findings?

a. Naltrexone
b. Physostigmine
c. Pralidoxime
d. Flumazenil

5-50. A 51-year-old male with chills, fever, and headache is thought to have "atypical" pneumonia. History reveals that he raises chickens and that approximately 2 weeks ago he lost a large number of them to an undiagnosed disease. The most likely diagnosis of this man's condition is

a. Anthrax
b. Q fever
c. Relapsing fever
d. Leptospirosis
e. Ornithosis (psittacosis)

Block 6

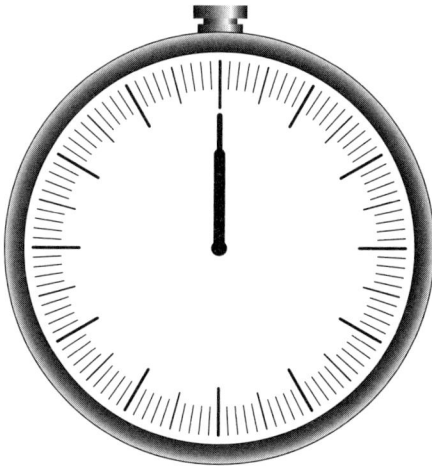

You have **60** minutes
to complete **50** questions.

BLOCK 6

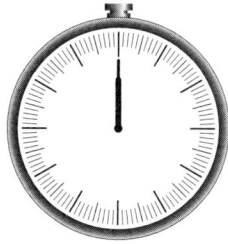

*YOU HAVE **60** MINUTES
TO COMPLETE **50** QUESTIONS.*

Questions

6-1. A 40-year-old male who works for the state as a highway and bridge designer becomes extremely anxious when he has to drive across any bridge—Which technique can best help him?

a. Habituation
b. Aversive conditioning
c. Stimulus control
d. Variable-ratio reinforcement
e. Systematic desensitization

6-2. A 48-year-old white female has what she feels is a suspicious lump in her breast, but a mammogram does not reveal any suspicious lesions. Truthful statements concerning potential pitfalls in management and diagnosis include

a. Assuming that mammography is "diagnostic"
b. Assuming that a radiographic lesion seen on mammography is the same as a palpable lesion
c. Not letting a negative or nonsuspicious mammogram influence the judgment of whether a palpable mass needs to be biopsied
d. Assuming that a benign aspiration cytology is definitive

Clinical Case (Questions 6-3 through 6-6)

Jane is a 75-year-old female who has taken medication for high blood pressure and high cholesterol for the past 10 years. One morning, upon awakening, she attempted to get up from her bed, only to find that she had difficulty walking, but didn't know why. When she tried to walk, her left leg collapsed beneath her. Jane couldn't understand why she was having so much difficulty waking, because she felt fine. Thinking that perhaps something was wrong, she edged her way across the floor to her telephone and promptly called for an ambulance. Jane hadn't noticed until now that her speech was slightly slurred. She was taken to the nearest emergency room for an evaluation.

Upon arriving in the emergency room, the staff noted that her face drooped on the left and that she persistently looked to her right side, and called a neurologist to see Jane. The neurologist tested Jane's language functions by asking her to name objects, repeat sentences, and write sentences, and thought that all of these tests were normal. Her speech was mildly slurred, and she had a right gaze preference. She would not cross the midline with her eyes when asked to look to the left, but instead, immediately returned her eyes to their right-sided gaze. When asked to raise her left hand, she raised her right hand. The neurologist asked Jane if her left hand belonged to her and she replied "no, it's yours." When asked to fill in the numbers of a clock, Jane put numbers 1 through 12 on the right side of the clock. When asked to bisect a line, she placed the perpendicular line on the right side. She did not blink to hand waving in the temporal visual field of her left eye, and the nasal visual field of her right eye. Other cranial nerves were normal, except for a left facial droop which spared the forehead. Her left arm and leg were markedly weak and the muscle tone was flaccid (floppy). All reflexes were depressed on the left side and normal on the right. The neurologist thought that all sensory modalities were depressed on the left side. The neurologist ordered a CT scan of Jane's head, and admitted her to the hospital for further work-up and treatment.

6-3. What kind of neurologic deficits does Jane have?

a. Left hemiparesis, hemineglect, left homonymous hemianopsia, left hemisensory loss
b. Left hemiparesis, right superior quadrantanopsia
c. Left hemiparesis, left hemisensory loss, hemineglect, left superior quadrantanopsia
d. Left hemisensory loss, hemineglect, bitemporal hemianopsia
e. Left hemisensory loss, hemineglect, left superior quadrantanopsia

6-4. Where in the nervous system has the damage occurred?

a. Left temporal and parietal lobes
b. Right frontal and temporal lobes
c. Right frontal and parietal lobes
d. Left frontal and parietal lobes
e. Left occipital lobe

6-5. If this damage was caused by a stroke, which artery became occluded?

a. Right anterior cerebral artery
b. Left anterior cerebral artery
c. Right posterior cerebral artery
d. Right middle cerebral artery
e. Left middle cerebral artery

6-6. Damage to which fibers caused Jane's inability to blink in response to the hand waving in her left temporal visual field?

a. Left facial nerve
b. Right oculomotor nerve
c. Left optic nerve
d. Optic chiasm
e. Right optic radiations

6-7. A 69-year-old male presents with urinary frequency, nocturia, dribbling, and difficulty in starting and stopping urination. Rectal examination reveals the prostate to be enlarged, firm, and rubbery. A needle biopsy reveals increased numbers of glandular elements and stromal tissue. The glands are found to have a double layer of epithelial cells. Prominent nuclei or back-to-back glands are not seen. What is the most likely diagnosis?

a. Acute prostatitis
b. Chronic bacterial prostatitis
c. Granulomatous prostatitis
d. Benign prostatic hyperplasia
e. Prostatic adenocarcinoma

6-8. A 28-year-old female succumbed after an 8-month course of severe dyspnea, fatigue, and cyanosis that followed an uneventful delivery of a healthy infant. At necropsy, small atheromas were present in the large and small branches of the pulmonary arteries. Which of the following findings can be predicted in the histologic slides of the lungs?

a. Diffuse hemorrhage and infarctions
b. Diffuse alveolar hyaline membranes
c. Severe atelectasis and edema
d. Marked medial hypertrophy of pulmonary arterioles
e. Multiple pulmonary emboli

6-9. A 48-year-old male living in an underdeveloped country presents with pain in the left side of his face. Physical examination reveals a large, indurated area involving the left side of his jaw with multiple sinuses draining pus. This draining material contains a few scattered small yellow granules. This lesion is most likely caused by an infection with

a. *Streptococcus pyogenes*
b. *Borrelia vincentii*
c. *Corynebacterium diphtheriae*
d. *Klebsiella rhinoscleromatis*
e. *Actinomyces israelii*

6-10. A 62-year-old male with hepatic failure secondary to cirrhosis develops a pungent odor in his breath (fetor hepaticus). He is also noted to have marked ascites, gynecomastia, asterixis, and palmar erythema. His serum ammonia levels are found to be elevated. This patient's gynecomastia is the result of

a. Decreased synthesis of albumin
b. Defective metabolism of the urea cycle
c. Deranged bilirubin metabolism
d. Impaired estrogen metabolism
e. The formation of mercaptans in gut

6-11. A 24-year-old female presents with severe pain during menses (dysmenorrhea). To treat her symptoms you advise her to take indomethacin in the hopes that it will reduce her pain by interfering with the production of

a. Bradykinin
b. Histamine
c. Leukotrienes
d. Phospholipase A_2
e. Prostaglandin F_2

6-12. A 59-year-old male with a history of rheumatic heart disease is found to have atrial fibrillation (AF), for which he is treated with digoxin. Treatment with digoxin converts his AF to normal sinus rhythm and most likely results in a decrease in which of the following?

a. The length of the refractory period
b. The velocity of shortening of the cardiac muscle
c. Conduction velocity in the atrioventricular (AV) node
d. The atrial maximum diastolic resting potential

6-13. A 23-year-old, semiconscious male is brought to the emergency room following an automobile accident. He is tachypneic (breathing rapidly) and cyanotic (blue lips and nail beds). The right lower anterolateral thoracic wall reveals a small laceration and flailing (moving inward as the rest of the thoracic cage expands during inspiration). Air does not appear to move into or out of the wound and it is assumed that the pleura has not been penetrated. After the patient is placed on immediate positive pressure endotracheal respiration, his cyanosis clears and the abnormal movement of the chest wall disappears. Radiographic examination confirms fractures of the fourth through eighth ribs in the right anterior axillary line and of the fourth through sixth ribs at the right costochondral junction. There is no evidence that bony fragments have penetrated the lungs or of pneumothorax (collapsed lung).

In this patient, the initial cyanosis is a result of

a. Bilateral inability of the pleural cavity to expand
b. Inability of the right chest wall to expand the thoracic cavity
c. Paralysis of the right hemidiaphragm
d. Paralysis of the thoracic musculature

6-14. A 45-year-old male has decreased libido and erectile dysfunction. He has noted increasing pigmentation. He has developed liver disease and arthropathy recently. The next best diagnostic test is

a. Serum TSH
b. Serum calcium
c. Serum prolactin
d. Serum ferritin
e. Serum gastrin

6-15. A 7-year-old male presents with bilateral swelling around his eyes. His parents state that this child's eyes have become "puffy" over the past several weeks, and his urine has become cocoa-colored. Physical examination reveals bilateral periorbital edema, but peripheral edema is not found. He is afebrile, and his blood pressure is slightly elevated. A urinary dipstick reveals mild proteinuria, while microscopic examination of his urine reveals hematuria with red blood cell casts. Laboratory tests reveal increased ASO titers and decreased serum C3 levels, but C2 and C4 levels are normal. A throat swab for *Streptococcus* is negative. A microscopic section from his kidney reveals increased numbers of cells within the glomeruli. An electron microscopic section of his kidney reveals large electron-dense deposits in the glomeruli that are located between the basement membrane and the podocytes. The foot processes of the podocytes are otherwise unremarkable. Which one of the following renal diseases most likely produced the abnormalities in this young boy?

a. Acute post-streptococcal glomerulonephritis
b. Focal segmental glomerulonephritis
c. Focal segmental glomerulosclerosis
d. Membranous glomerulonephritis
e. Minimal change disease

6-16. A 38-year-old industrial foundry worker who has been chronically exposed to heavy metal vapors has developed a radiographic pattern of pulmonary "honeycombing." Which of the following heavy metals is most likely responsible?

a.   Cobalt
b.   Lead
c.   Cadmium
d.   Mercury
e.   Arsenic

6-17. An uncircumcised 49-year-old male presents with the sudden onset of severe pain in the distal portion of his penis. The emergency room physician examines the patient and finds that the foreskin is retracted but cannot be rolled back over the glans penis. The ER physician calls the urologist who performs an emergency resection of this patient's foreskin. What is the most likely diagnosis?

a.   Balanoposthitis
b.   Bladder exstrophy
c.   Epispadia
d.   Hypospadia
e.   Paraphimosis

6-18. A 26-year-old female in the third trimester of her first pregnancy develops persistent headaches and swelling of her legs and face. Early during her pregnancy a physical examination was unremarkable, however, now her blood pressure is 170/105 mmHg, and a urinalysis reveals slight proteinuria.

What is the most likely diagnosis?

a.   Eclampsia
b.   Gestational trophoblastic disease
c.   Nephritic syndrome
d.   Nephrotic syndrome
e.   Preeclampsia

6-19. A newborn infant had severe respiratory problems. Over the next few days, it was observed that the baby had severe muscle problems, demonstrated little development, and had neurological problems. A liver biopsy revealed a very low level of acetyl CoA carboxylase, but normal levels of the enzymes of glycolysis, gluconeogenesis, the citric acid cycle, and the pentose phosphate pathway. What is the most likely cause of the infant's respiratory problems?

a.   Low levels of phosphatidyl choline
b.   Biotin deficiency
c.   Ketoacidosis
d.   High levels of citrate
e.   Glycogen depletion

6-20. A 36-year-old male has been experiencing intense pressure to be more productive at work. This has resulted in his becoming extremely anxious, which makes it very difficult for him to function effectively. He wishes to keep his job. Physical examination and blood chemistries are normal. He is given diazepam, which diminishes his anxiety and allows him to concentrate on his work. What is this drug's mechanism of action?

a. It directly opens the Cl⁻ channel of the GABA receptor
b. It increases the frequency of opening of the Cl⁻ channel of the GABA receptor
c. It prolongs the duration of opening of the Cl⁻ channel of the GABA receptor

6-21. A 23-year-old female presents with progressive bilateral loss of central vision. You obtain a detailed family history from this patient and produce the associated pedigree (dark circles or squares indicate affected individuals). Which of the following transmission patterns is most consistent with this patient's family history?

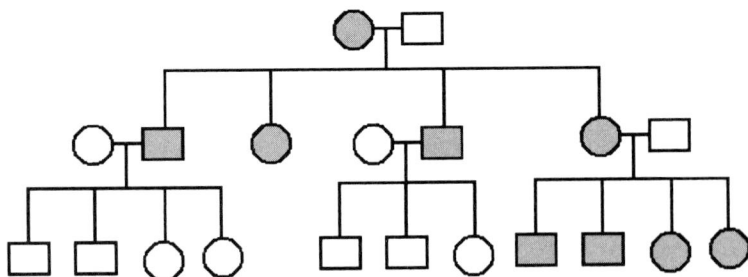

a. Autosomal recessive
b. Autosomal dominant
c. X-linked recessive
d. X-linked dominant
e. Mitochondrial

6-22. A 20-year-old male presents in the emergency room with a lymphoma involving the mediastinum that is producing respiratory distress. The lymphocytes are most likely to have cell surface markers characteristic of which of the following?

a. B cells
b. T cells
c. Macrophages
d. Dendritic reticulum cells
e. Langerhans cells

6-23. A 19-year-old female presents with oligomenorrhea. Physical examination reveals an obese young female with acne and increased facial hair. A pelvic examination is essentially within normal limits, excluding the adnexal regions which could not be palpated secondary to obesity. Work-up reveals increased serum levels of luteinizing hormones (LH), androgens, and estrogens, normal amounts of thyroid stimulating hormone (TSH) and prolactin, and decreased levels of follicle stimulating hormone (FSH). Exploration of this individual's abdomen would most likely reveal

a. A benign ovarian neoplasm
b. A malignant ovarian neoplasm
c. Bilateral atrophy of the ovaries (streak ovaries)
d. Bilateral enlargement of the ovaries with multiple subcortical cysts
e. Endometriosis of the ovaries and the fallopian tubes

6-24. A 25-year-old female presents with a three year history of infertility. Obtaining a history you find out that her cycles have averaged consistently about 33 days in length, and the length of menstruation has also been a constant 4 days in length. You decide to take an endometrial biopsy approximately 2 to 3 days after the predicted time of ovulation. If the cause of her infertility relates to inadequate functioning of the corpus luteum, then biopsies of her endometrium would most likely reveal

a. Non-secretory endometrium with mild hyperplasia
b. Chronologic day and histologic appearance asynchrony
c. Inactive glands within predecidualized stroma
d. Atrophic endometrium (glands and stroma)
e. Secretory glands mixed with proliferative glands

6-25. A 23-year-old male with full-blown AIDS is noted to be severely neutropenic. Which of the following abnormalities is most likely to be seen on further investigation?

a. Macrocytic anemia
b. Normal CD4 lymphocyte count
c. Thrombocytopenia
d. Lymphocytosis
e. Hypocellular bone marrow

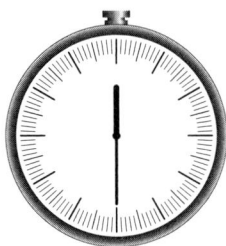

YOU SHOULD HAVE COMPLETED APPROXIMATELY
25 QUESTIONS AND HAVE 30 MINUTES REMAINING.

Clinical Case (Questions 6-26 through 6-29)

June is a 65-year-old female who was previously healthy. One day, while taking a walk in the park, she noticed her right fingers twitching, then her right hand, then her arm and shoulder, followed by a march of twitches down her leg. She did not remember any more than this, because she lost consciousness. An onlooker saw her drop to the ground and deviate her neck backward, while making a high-pitched noise. Then, both of her arms and legs began to jerk for approximately 1 to 2 minutes, then stopped abruptly. She had lost control of her bladder during this event. When the onlooker attempted to speak to June to ask her if she was okay, she was unresponsive. The onlooker called an ambulance, which brought June to the nearest hospital.

A doctor met June at the emergency room entrance, and asked her what had happened. By this time, June was slightly drowsy, but able to answer questions appropriately. Her speech was fluent and grammatically correct. She knew the month, but not the day of the week, or where she was. She moved the left side of her body better than her right, but had too much difficulty following commands for an effective motor examination. The remainder of her examination was normal. The doctor ordered a CT of June's head and drew some blood.

6-26. From which area of the brain did June's seizure begin?

a. Left precentral gyrus
b. Right precentral gyrus
c. Right temporal lobe
d. Left temporal lobe
e. Thalamus

6-27. What could account for June's loss of consciousness following the seizure?

a. Involvement of the reticular activating system
b. Head trauma
c. Bilateral post-ictal suppression
d. Thalamic involvement
e. Brain hemorrhage from the seizure

6-28. The "march" of twitching which June experienced can be explained by

a. Proximity of the body part to the spinal cord
b. Proximity of the body part to the cerebral cortex
c. Somatotopic representation within brainstem
d. Somatotopic representation within the basal ganglia
e. Somatotopic representation within the precentral gyrus

6-29. Which cell type is the predominant cause of the seizure?

a. Basket cell
b. Purkinje cell
c. Stellate cell
d. Schwann cell
e. Pyramidal cell

6-30. A 21-year-old college student complained of malaise, low-grade fever, and a harsh cough, but not of muscle aches and pains. An x-ray revealed a diffuse interstitial pneumonia in the left lobes of the lung. The WBC count was normal. The student has been ill for a week.

Based on the information given, the most likely diagnosis is

a. *Mycoplasma* pneumonia
b. Pneumococcal pneumonia
c. Staphylococcal pneumonia
d. Influenza
e. Legionellosis

6-31. A 47-year-old male has had a headache and experienced impotence for the past 2 months. A likely hormonal profile would be

a. Low testosterone, high LH, and low prolactin
b. Low testosterone, low LH, and low prolactin
c. Low testosterone, high LH, and high prolactin
d. Normal testosterone, normal LH, and normal prolactin
e. Low testosterone, low LH, and high prolactin

6-32. A 45-year-old male with an artificial heart valve is given oral Coumadin (Warfarin) to prevent the formation of thrombi on his artificial valve. Which combination of laboratory tests is most likely to be found in this individual?

	Tourniquet test	Bleeding time	Platelet count	PTT	PT
a.	Positive	Prolonged	Normal	Normal	Normal
b.	Normal	Normal	Normal	Prolonged	Normal
c.	Positive	Prolonged	Decreased	Normal	Normal
d.	Normal	Normal	Normal	Normal	Prolonged
e.	Normal	Prolonged	Normal	Prolonged	Normal

6-33. A 5-year-old Egyptian male receives a course of the antibiotic sulfamethoxazole as prophylaxis for recurrent urinary tract infections. Although he was previously healthy and well-nourished, he becomes progressively ill and presents to your office with pallor and irritability. A blood count shows that he is severely anemic with jaundice due to hemolysis of red blood cells.

The most likely diagnosis would be

a. Anemia because of sickle cell anemia
b. Anemia due to nutritional deficiency
c. Drug reaction due to Rh antigen incompatibility
d. Drug reaction due to glucose-6-phosphate dehydrogenase deficiency
e. Anemia because of β-thalassemia

6-34. A jaundiced one-day-old premature infant with an elevated free bilirubin is seen in the premature-baby nursery. The mother received an antibiotic combination preparation containing sulfamethizole for a urinary tract infection (UTI) one week before delivery. You suspect that the infant's findings are caused by the sulfonamide because of the following mechanism:

a. Enhanced synthesis of bilirubin
b. Competition between the sulfonamide and bilirubin for binding sites on albumin
c. Inhibition of bilirubin degradation
d. Inhibition of urinary excretion of bilirubin

6-35. A young male is being evaluated for developmental delay, mild autism, and mental retardation. Physical examination reveals the boy to have large, everted ears, and a long face with a large mandible. He is also found to have macroorchidism (large testes) and extensive work-up reveals multiple tandem repeats of the nucleotide sequence CGG in his DNA. Which one of the following is the most likely diagnosis for this patient?

a. Fragile X syndrome
b. Huntington's chorea
c. Myotonic dystrophy
d. Spinal-bulbar muscular atrophy
e. Ataxia-telangiectasia

6-36. A 31-year-old male is infertile. His medical history reveals that he has Kartagener's syndrome. Why is he infertile?

a. Oligospermia
b. Asthenospermia
c. Absence of the vas deferens
d. Epididymal obstruction
e. Undescended testes

Clinical Case (Questions 6-37 through 6-40)

Mike is a 35-year-old male who had optic neuritis (an inflammation of the optic nerve causing blurred vision) several years before. He was told that he had a 50 percent chance of eventually developing multiple sclerosis, a degenerative disease of the CNS white matter. One day, he noticed that he had double vision and felt weak on his right side. Although he noted that the symptoms were becoming steadily worse throughout the day, he attributed this to stress from his job as a stockbroker, and in order to relax, he decided to take a drive in his car. While he was driving, his vision became steadily worse. As he was about to pull over to the side of the road, he saw two trees on the right side of the road. Uncertain which was the actual image, he attempted to place his right foot on the break pedal. Mike suddenly realized that he was unable to lift his right leg, and his car collided with the tree. A pedestrian on the side of the road called EMS, and Mike was brought to a nearby emergency room.

A neurologist was called to see Mike because the emergency room physicians thought he may have had a stroke, despite his young age. The neurologist spoke to Mike, then examined him. He found that his left eye was deviated to the left and down. When he attempted to look to his right, his right eye moved normally, but his left eye was unable to move further to the right than the midline. His left pupil was dilated and did not contract to light from a penlight. His left eyelid drooped, and he had difficulty raising it. In addition, the right side of his mouth remained motionless when he attempted to smile, but his forehead was symmetric when he raised his eyebrows. Mike's right arm and leg were markedly weak. The neurologist told Mike that he wasn't certain that this was necessarily a stroke, but admitted him to the hospital for observation and tests.

6-37. A lesion in which nerve caused Mike's double vision?

a. Optic nerve
b. Oculomotor nerve
c. Cervical sympathetic fibers
d. Trochlear nerve
e. Abducens nerve

6-38. Damage to nerves innervating which eye muscles cause Mike's eye to be deviated toward the left side and down?

a. Superior rectus, superior oblique, inferior rectus, inferior oblique
b. Superior rectus, inferior rectus, inferior oblique, lateral rectus
c. Superior rectus, inferior rectus, inferior oblique, medial rectus
d. Lateral rectus, superior oblique, medial rectus, inferior rectus
e. Lateral rectus, superior oblique, inferior oblique, medial rectus

6-39. Where in the nervous system did the damage occur?

a. Left frontal lobe
b. Right frontal lobe
c. Left eye
d. Cervical spinal cord
e. Midbrain

6-40. Damage to which fibers caused the enlarged, unreactive left pupil?

a. Medial longitudinal fasciculus
b. Frontal or pontine eye fields
c. Edinger-Westphal nucleus or pre-ganglionic parasympathetic fibers
d. Trochlear nerve
e. Cervical sympathetic fibers

6-41. A 19-year-old female whose roommate is being treated for depression decides that she is also depressed and secretly takes her roommate's pills "as directed on the bottle" for several days. One night, she makes herself a snack of chicken liver paté and bleu cheese, accompanied by a glass of red wine. She soon develops headache, nausea, and palpitations. She goes to the ED, where her blood pressure is found to be 200/110 mmHg. What antidepressant did she take?

a. Sertraline
b. Phenelzine
c. Nortriptyline
d. Trazodone
e. Fluoxetine

6-42. A 52-year-old white female with breast cancer on adjuvant therapy presents with back pain that intensifies upon movement, and pain over the L-1 vertebral body when she coughs, and that radiates down her left lower extremity to her leg and foot. The most likely etiology of this disorder is

a. Paraneoplastic disorder
b. Trauma to the lumbar disc
c. Muscular spasm of the intercostal muscles
d. Possible spinal cord compression

6-43. A 65-year-old female has experienced a slow onset of rheumatoid arthritis in her hands and shoulder joints over the past ten years. Treatment has slowed the progress of the disease. Her arthritis is not severe and she stays active, but she has scheduled an office visit for help with what she admits to be stress problems and anxiety. Even before her examination you suspect that the principal source of her psychosocial stress is

a. Loss of coping skills
b. Loss of self-esteem
c. Physical disability
d. Uncontrollable bouts of pain
e. Concern for her future

6-44. A 31-year-old female presents with fever, intermittent severe pain in her left upper quadrant of her abdomen, and painful lesions involving her fingers and nailbeds. History reveals that she had acute rheumatic fever as a child, and when she was around 20 years of age she developed a new cardiac murmur. At the present time one of three blood cultures submitted to the hospital lab grows out a particular organism. Which one of the following is most likely to be that organism?

a. *Staphylococcus aureus*
b. α-Hemolytic viridans streptococci
c. *Candida* species
d. Group A streptococci
e. *Pseudomonas* species

6-45. An infant is brought in by his mother, who says that his skin tastes salty. With time this patient's pancreas will be expected to undergo progressive fibrosis with atrophy of the exocrine glands and cystic dilatation of the ducts. The basic abnormality in this infant involves

a. Decreased synthesis of surface receptor
b. Decreased intracellular cAMP
c. Decreased glycosylated chloride channel
d. Increased phosphorylation of chloride channel
e. Increased ductal secretion of water

6-46. A 59-year-old female presents with difficulty swallowing, ptosis, and diplopia. Which of the following is most consistent with these symptoms?

a. Antibodies to the acetylcholine receptor
b. Antibodies to the microvasculature of skeletal muscle
c. Lack of lactate production during ischemic exercise
d. Rhabdomyolysis
e. Corticosteroid therapy

6-47. A 6-year-old female presented to the clinic with scaly patches on the scalp. Primary smears and culture of the skin and hair were negative. A few weeks later, she returned and was found to have inflammatory lesions. The hair fluoresced under Wood's light and primary smears of skin and hair contained septate hyphae. On speaking with the parents, it was discovered that there were several pets in the household. Which of the following is the most likely agent?

a. *Microsporum audouini*
b. *Microsporum canis*
c. *Trichophyton tonsurans*
d. *Trichophyton rubrum*
e. *Epidermophyton floccosum*

6-48. A 16-year-old male presents without pubertal development and development of secondary sexual characteristics. He cannot smell (anosmia). The baseline testosterone and the LH response to LHRH most likely are

a. Low testosterone and normal LHRH response
b. Normal testosterone and normal LHRH response
c. High testosterone and normal LHRH response
d. Low testosterone and no LHRH response
e. Low testosterone and exaggerated LHRH response

6-49. A 21-year-old male college athlete presents with a nagging cough and a 20 pound weight loss. In addition to the chronic cough and weight loss, his main symptoms consist of fever, night sweats, and chest pains. Examination of his sputum reveals the presence of rare acid-fast organisms. His symptoms are most likely due to an infection with

a. *Klebsiella pneumoniae*
b. *Legionella pneumophila*
c. *Mycobacterium avium-intracellulare*
d. *Mycobacterium tuberculosis*
e. *Mycoplasma pneumonia*

6-50. A 15-year-old male has a lack of pubic hair growth. He also informs you that his voice has not yet deepened, and he has no interest in sexual activity. He is an only child. Blood drawn reveals a very high testosterone level. What is the problem?

a. Low FSH and LH
b. High FSH and LH
c. Androgen insensitivity
d. Hyperthyroidism
e. XXY karyotype

BLOCK 7

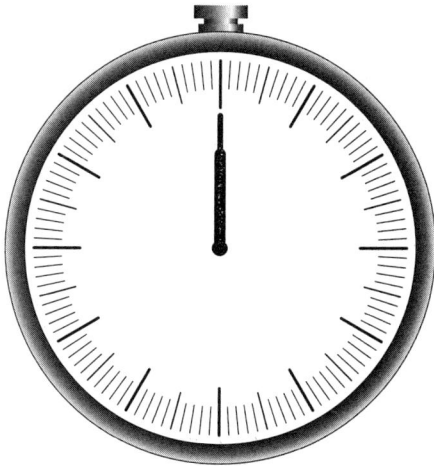

YOU HAVE **60** MINUTES
TO COMPLETE **50** QUESTIONS.

BLOCK 7

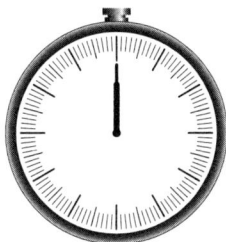

YOU HAVE *60* MINUTES
TO COMPLETE *50* QUESTIONS.

Questions

7-1. A child is referred for evaluation of developmental delay and unusual behavior. On examination, the physician notes loose joints, large ears, prominent jaw, and large testes for age.

This child's condition is most likely to be a

a. Sequence
b. Syndrome
c. Disruption
d. Single birth defect
e. Deformation

7-2. A 10-year-old female asthmatic patient receives cromolyn daily as part of her therapeutic regimen. Cromolyn functions primarily as

a. A β_2-agonist
b. A histamine$_1$ (H$_1$) receptor antagonist
c. An anticholinergic
d. An inhibitor of mediator release

7-3. A 71-year-old female presents with the sudden onset of severe lower back pain. Physical examination reveals severe kyphosis, while an x-ray of her back reveals a compression fracture of a vertebral body in the lumbar area along with marked thinning of the bones. Serum calcium, phosphorus, alkaline phosphatase, and parathyroid hormone levels are all within normal limits. Her bone changes are most likely due to

a. Osteopetrosis
b. Osteoporosis
c. Osteomalacia
d. Osteitis fibrosa cystica
e. Osteitis deformans

7-4. A 47-year-old male presents with pain in the mid-portion of his chest. The pain is associated with eating and swallowing food. Endoscopic examination reveals an ulcerated area in the lower portion of his esophagus. Histologic sections of tissue taken from this area reveal an ulceration of the esophageal mucosa that is filled with blood, fibrin, proliferating blood vessels, and proliferating fibroblasts. Mitoses are easily found, and most of the cells have prominent nucleoli. Which one of the following correctly describes this ulcerated area?

a. Caseating granulomatous inflammation
b. Dysplastic epithelium
c. Granulation tissue
d. Squamous cell carcinoma
e. Noncaseating granulomatous inflammation

7-5. An 8-year-old male is found to have progressive corneal vascularization, deafness, notched incisors, and a flattened nose. The most likely cause of these changes is congenital infection by

a. Toxoplasma
b. Rubella
c. Cytomegalovirus
d. Herpes simplex virus
e. *Treponema pallidum*

Clinical Case (Questions 7-6 through 7-9)
Louise is an 86-year-old female who has had difficulty with high blood pressure, high cholesterol, diabetes, strokes, and blood clots in her legs for many years. One day, her grandson arrived at her apartment in a senior citizen center for his weekly visit, only to find her lying unconscious on the floor. He immediately called an ambulance to bring her to the nearest emergency room.

The paramedics in the ambulance gave Louise some medications, including glucose, but she did not awaken. She was brought to the nearest emergency room, where a physician was called to evaluate her. She was breathing on her own and had a pulse, but could not be aroused to any stimulus. Her arms and legs were stiff, and would not move in response to a painful stimulus. Her eyes moved in response to moving her head. Finally, in response to a very loud shout and pinch on the arm, she briefly opened her eyes, however she immediately shut them again. Further attempts to arouse Louise were unsuccessful. She was taken for a CT scan of her head, and then brought to an intensive care unit.

7-6. An acute stroke in which portion of the central nervous system could cause this situation?

a. Right frontal lobe
b. Left frontal lobe
c. Right temporal lobe
d. Pons and midbrain
e. Right occipital lobe

7-7. What is the cause of the stiffness in Louise's arms and legs?

a. Infarction of the corticospinal tracts bilaterally in the pons
b. Damage to the basal ganglia
c. Infarction of the precentral gyrus
d. Infarction of the internal capsules bilaterally
e. Thalamic infarction

7-8. Infarction of which artery may cause this picture?

a. Anterior cerebral artery
b. Middle cerebral artery
c. Anterior choroidal artery
d. Basilar artery
e. Lenticulostriate branches of the middle cerebral artery

7-9. If the stroke occurred in the brainstem, which region is most likely affected?

a. Facial nerve nucleus
b. Trochlear nerve nucleus
c. Reticular formation
d. Trigeminal system
e. Medial longitudinal fasciculus

7-10. A 55-year-old male has lung cancer in the right middle lobe. Syndromes H associated with the lung cancer include

a. Hypocalcemia
b. Hypocortisolemia
c. Hyperphosphatemia
d. Acromegaly

7-11. A 28-year-old female has had 2 days of abdominal pain and a positive pregnancy test. Her last menstrual period was 9 weeks ago. She reports no dysuria. She reports a history of two episodes of pelvic inflammatory disease. Which of these is the most likely cause of the abdominal pain?

a. Endometriosis
b. Urinary tract infection
c. Ectopic pregnancy
d. Placental abruption
e. Premenstrual syndrome

7-12. A 27-year-old female presents with headaches, muscle pain (myalgia), anorexia, nausea, and vomiting. She denies any history of drug or alcohol use, but upon further questioning she states that recently she has lost her taste for coffee and cigarettes. Physical examination reveals a slight yellow discoloration to her sclerae, while laboratory results indicate a serum bilirubin level of 1.8 mg/dL, and the aminotransferases (AST and ALT) levels are increased. These signs and symptoms are most consistent with a diagnosis of

a. Gilbert's syndrome
b. Chronic hepatitis
c. Amebic liver abscess
d. Acute viral hepatitis
e. Acute hepatic failure

7-13. A 36-year-old male presents because his skin has been darkening recently. You notice that his skin has a dark, somewhat bronze color. Work-up reveals signs of diabetes mellitus. His serum iron is found to be 1,150 μg/dL, and his transferrin saturation is 98 percent. A liver biopsy is performed and reveals extensive deposits of hemosiderin in the hepatocytes and Kupffer cells. What is your diagnosis?

a. Alpha-1-antitrypsin deficiency
b. Dubin-Johnson syndrome
c. Primary hemochromatosis
d. Reye's syndrome

7-14. A 27-year-old female has just returned from a trip to Southeast Asia. In the past 24 hours, she has developed shaking, chills, and a temperature of 104°F. A blood smear reveals *Plasmodium vivax*. Which of the following agents is the drug of choice?

a. Primaquine
b. Pyrimethamine
c. Quinacrine
d. Chloroquine
e. Chloroguanide

7-15. A 33-year-old female with an average menstrual cycle of 28 days comes in for a routine Pap smear. It has been 35 days since the start of her last menstrual period, and a vaginal smear reveals clumps of basophilic cells. You suspect:

a. She will begin menstruating in a few days
b. She will ovulate within a few days
c. Her serum progesterone levels are very low
d. There are detectable levels of hCG in her serum and urine
e. She is undergoing menopause

7-16. A 49-year-old female presents with signs of anemia, and states that every morning her urine is dark. Work-up reveals that her red blood cells lyse in vitro with acid (positive Ham's test). What is the best diagnosis for this patient?

a. Warm autoimmune hemolytic anemia
b. Paroxysmal nocturnal hemoglobinuria
c. Paroxysmal cold hemoglobinuria
d. Isoimmune hemolytic anemia
e. Cold agglutinin autoimmune hemolytic anemia

7-17. A 2-year-old male presents with repeated viral and fungal infections and tetany. Work-up reveals hypocalcemia and a marked impairment of cell-mediated immunity resulting from an absence of T cells. Because of these signs and symptoms, the diagnosis of DiGeorge's syndrome is made. Considering this diagnosis, the absence of T cells is a direct consequence of failure of which embryonic structure to develop?

a. Third pharyngeal pouch
b. Fourth pharyngeal pouch
c. Fifth pharyngeal pouch
d. Ultimobranchial body
e. Foramen cecum

7-18. A 22-year-old female marathon runner has had amenorrhea for 8 months. There has been no weight change, and her serum pregnancy test is negative. She has never been pregnant. Her menarche was at 13 years of age, and she had monthly menses until 8 months ago. Physical exam shows a female who is 66 inches tall, weighs 90 pounds, and is otherwise fully normal. Why does she have amenorrhea?

a. Hypothyroidism
b. Prolactinoma
c. Early menopause
d. Resistance to LH and follicle-stimulating hormone (FSH)
e. Excessive exercise

7-19. A comatose 27-year-old female is brought to the emergency room by paramedics, and the strong odor of bitter almonds is present. The differential diagnosis must include the possibility of poisoning by

a. Ethylene glycol
b. Carbon monoxide
c. Mercury
d. Cyanide
e. Methanol

7-20. A 21-year-old female presents because her urine has turned a brown color. She states that about two months ago her urine turned brown two days after a cold and stayed brown for about three days. At the current time a urinalysis reveals 2+ blood with red cells and red cell casts. Further laboratory tests include a complete blood count (CBC), serum electrolytes, BUN, creatinine, glucose, antinuclear antibodies (ANA), and serum complement levels (C3 and C4). All of these tests are within normal limits. Immunofluorescence examination of a renal biopsy from this patient reveals the presence of large, irregular deposits of IgA/C3 in the mesangium. A linear staining pattern is not found. What is the most likely diagnosis for this patient?

a. Berger's disease
b. Focal segmental glomerulosclerosis
c. Goodpasture's disease
d. Lipoid nephrosis
e. Membranoproliferative glomerulonephritis

7-21. A 28-year-old male presents with widespread ecchymoses and bleeding gums. Physical examination reveals enlargement of his spleen and liver. Laboratory examination of his peripheral blood reveals a normochromic, normocytic anemia, along with a decreased number of platelets, and increased number of white blood cells. Coagulation studies reveal prolonged prothrombin and partial thromboplastin times, and increased fibrinogen degradation products. Examination of his bone marrow reveals the presence of numerous granular-appearing blast cells with numerous Auer rods. These immature cells comprise about 38 percent of the nucleated cells in the marrow. The diagnosis for this patient is

a. Acute erythroid leukemia
b. Acute lymphoblastic leukemia
c. Acute monocytic leukemia
d. Acute myelomonocytic leukemia
e. Acute progranulocytic leukemia

7-22. During a routine physical examination A 60-year-old white male is found to have a 5 cm pulsatile mass in his abdomen. Angiography reveals a marked dilatation of his aorta distal to his renal arteries. This aneurysm is most likely the result of

a. Atherosclerosis
b. A congenital defect
c. Hypertension
d. A previous syphilitic infection
e. Trauma

Clinical Case (Questions 7-23 through 7-26)

Julie is a 29-year-old office worker with diabetes, who awoke one morning with the inability to close her left eye, and a left facial droop. Her left eye felt a bit dry, as well. She had run out of sick days, and hoping that the problem would go away, went to work. After several co-workers noticed that her face was drooping, and that she was especially sensitive to loud noises on her left side, they convinced her to go to the nearest emergency room in order to make sure that she did not have a stroke.

She was examined right away in the emergency room, because of her age. The doctor noted immediately that her mouth drooped on the left side. Her left eye was slightly closed. He tested her speech and mental status, which were normal, other than some slight slurring of her speech. Her vision and eye movements were also normal. Sensation and jaw movement were also normal, but when she was asked to wiggle her eyebrows, only the right side of her forehead moved. When asked to close her eyes tightly, and not allow him to open her eyes, her right eye would not open, but her left eye could not oppose the force. She was not able to hold air in her cheeks when asked to hold her breath, and when asked to smile, only the right side of her mouth elevated. She was very sensitive to noise on her left side. When asked to protrude her tongue, it did not deviate to either side, but if she closed her eyes and sugar-water was placed on the left side of the anterior portion of her tongue, she could not identify it. The remainder of her examination was normal. A nurse asked if a head CT should be ordered in order to look for a stroke or tumor, but the doctor said that it was not necessary. He told Julie that he would draw some blood, and give her a medication to take for a while.

7-23. Assuming that the doctor was correct, and that this is not a stroke, where in the nervous system has the damage occurred?

a. Buccinator muscle
b. Trigeminal nerve
c. Facial nerve
d. Glossopharyngeal nerve
e. Hypoglossal nerve

7-24. Julie's facial weakness is characteristic of

a. A muscle lesion
b. A lesion of the internal capsule
c. A superior brainstem lesion
d. An upper motor neuron seventh nerve lesion
e. A lower motor neuron seventh nerve lesion

7-25. Damage to which area may have produced the defect in taste in the anterior two thirds of her tongue?

a. Intermediate nerve
b. Glossopharyngeal nerve
c. Lingual nerve
d. Facial nerve, distal to the chorda tympani nerve
e. Facial nerve, proximal to the chorda tympani nerve

7-26. Assuming that Julie had no prior problems with her ears or cochlear nerve, damage to the nerve supply of which muscle could cause the sensitivity to or distortion of noises?

a. Digastric
b. Platysma
c. Buccinator
d. Geniohyoid
e. Stapedius

.

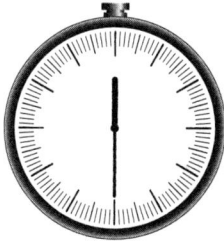

YOU SHOULD HAVE COMPLETED APPROXIMATELY 25 QUESTIONS AND HAVE 30 MINUTES REMAINING.

7-27. You are asked to see a 45-year-old male patient who is complaining of frequent chest pains. As you enter the examining room, the patient is sobbing and blurts out, "My father died just like this 2 years ago." Your next step should be to

a. Reassure him that his pain is not related to his father's illness
b. Get more information on how his father's pain manifested itself
c. Order an emergency electrocardiogram
d. Introduce yourself and inquire about family history of heart disease
e. Ask a sufficient number of direct medical questions to establish that this is not an emergency

7-28. A 30-year-old male patient was seen by the Emergency Service and reported a two-week history of a penile ulcer. He noted that this ulcer did not hurt. Which one of the following conclusions/actions is most valid?

a. Draw blood for a herpes antibody test
b. Perform a dark field examination of the lesion
c. Prescribe acyclovir for primary genital herpes
d. Even if treated, the lesion will remain for months
e. Failure to treat the patient will have no untoward effect as this is a self-limiting infection

7-29. A 66-year-old white female with a known history of small cell lung cancer comes to your office because of engorgement of her neck veins on the right side and over her chest wall. She also has cyanosis of the extremities, facial edema, and difficulty with her mentation. Her diagnosis is most likely

a. Congestive heart failure
b. Lymphatic obstruction of the upper body
c. Superior vena cava syndrome
d. Deep venous thrombosis

7-30. A 23-year-old female develops the sudden onset of congestive heart failure. Her condition rapidly deteriorates and she dies in heart failure. At autopsy, patchy interstitial infiltrates composed mainly of lymphocytes are found, some of which surround individual myoytes. The most likely cause of this patient's heart failure is

a. Viral myocarditis
b. Bacterial myocarditis
c. Giant cell myocarditis
d. Hypersensitivity myocarditis
e. Beriberi

7-31. A 23-year-old female presents with the recent onset of a vaginal discharge. Physical examination reveals multiple clear vesicles on her vulva and vagina. A smear of material obtained from one of these vesicles reveals several multinucleated giant cell with intranuclear inclusions and ground glass nuclei. These vesicles are most likely the result of an infection with

a. Cytomegalovirus (CMV)
b. Herpes simplex virus (HSV)
c. Human papillomavirus (HPV)
d. *Candida albicans*
e. *Trichomonas vaginalis*

7-32. A 65-year-old female receives digoxin and furosemide for CHF. After several months, she develops nausea and vomiting. Serum K⁺ is 2.5 mEq/L. Electrocardiogram (EKG) reveals an AV conduction defect. What cellular effect is causing these new findings?

a. Increased intracellular K
b. Increased intracellular guanosine 3'5'-cyclic monophosphate (cGMP)
c. Increased intracellular Ca
d. Increased intracellular norepinephrine
e. Increased intracellular nitric oxide (NO)

7-33. A 28-year-old female has amenorrhea and galactorrhea, after beginning a new medication recently. The most likely medication is

a. Haloperidol
b. Lisinopril
c. Fluoxetine
d. Amitriptyline
e. Buspirone

7-34. A 52-year-old female is having hot flashes. You suspect menopause. Which of the findings below would confirm your diagnosis?

a. Normal androgen level
b. Normal or low estrogen level
c. Normal prolactin level
d. High FSH and LH levels
e. High androgen level

7-35. A 37-year-old male with a history of alcohol abuse was seen in the emergency room complaining of stomach cramps in the region of the umbilicus. He reported several recent incidents of vomiting that contained no noticeable blood, although he had in the past vomited bright red blood. He insisted that he had been on the wagon for the past several months. Physical examination revealed a mass about the umbilicus with indications of periumbilical peritoneal inflammation. His white blood cell count was high and he had a temperature of 39.4°C (103°F). He was admitted to the surgical service for emergency reduction of an umbilical hernia with suspected strangulation.

The crampy abdominal pain referred to the umbilical region and knowledge of peritoneal structure would lead the examining physician to suspect that the strangulated section of gut was most likely the

a. Ascending colon
b. Descending colon
c. Small intestine
d. Sigmoid colon
e. Stomach

7-36. A 30-year-old female stored her contact lenses in tap water. She noticed deterioration of vision and visited an ophthalmologist who diagnosed her with severe retinitis. Culture of the water as well as vitreous fluid would most likely reveal

a. Naegleria
b. *Pneumocystis*
c. *Acanthamoeba*
d. *Babesia*
e. *Entamoeba coli*

7-37. A 46-year-old female undergoes an abdominal hysterectomy for a "fibroid" uterus. The surgeon requests a frozen section on the tumor, which is deferred because of the lesion's degree of cellularity. Which of the following criteria will be used by the pathologist in determining benignancy versus malignancy in permanent sections?

a. Mitotic rate
b. Cell pleomorphism
c. Cell necrosis
d. Nucleocytoplasmic (NC) ratio
e. Tumor size

Clinical Case (Questions 7-38 through 7-41)

Herb, a 62-year-old male, who has smoked two packs of cigarettes per day for 35 years, was suffering from a chronic cough that was attributed to a smoking habit by his physician. One day, Herb noticed that his right eyelid drooped slightly, and that his right pupil was smaller than the left. He also noticed that the inner side of his right hand was numb, and that he had begun to drop things from his right hand. He had no other symptoms. Herb consulted his physician who directed him to a neurologist.

The neurologist noted that although the right pupil was smaller than the left, it was still reactive to light. Although Herb's right eyelid drooped slightly, he could close his eyes tightly when asked to do so. The neurologist noted that Herb did not sweat on the right side of his face. He was unable to feel a pinprick on the inner surface of his right hand, and his right triceps and hand muscles were weak.

7-38. Where in the nervous system has damage occurred?

a. Left oculomotor nerve
b. Right oculomotor nerve
c. Nucleus of Edinger-Westphal
d. Sympathetic fibers coursing from the hypothalamus to the intermediolateral cell column
e. Parasympathetic fibers coursing from the nucleus of Edinger-Westphal

7-39. Herb's small pupil is due to

a. Unopposed action of muscles with parasympathetic innervation
b. Unopposed action of muscles with sympathetic innervation
c. Both sympathetic and parasympathetic damage
d. A lesion in the nucleus of the third nerve
e. A lesion in distal branches of the trochlear nerve

7-40. Why was Herb able to close his eye tightly, despite a drooping eyelid?

a. The facial nerve does not innervate muscles mediating eye closure
b. The facial nerve is only partially affected
c. The facial nerve is unaffected by this lesion
d. The trigeminal nerve compensates for eye closure
e. This lesion only affects involuntary eye closure

7-41. Which pair of neurotransmitters is involved in the pathway that has been damaged?

a. Substance P and acetylcholine
b. Norepinephrine and epinephrine
c. 5-HT and GABA
d. GABA and acetylcholine
e. Acetylcholine and norepinephrine

7-42. A 21-year-old HIV-positive male presents with malaise, fever, and increasing lymph nodes in his right cervical region. A microscopic section from one of the enlarged lymph nodes that is stained with an acid-fast stain reveals the presence of numerous ("too many to count") acid-fast organisms. Granulomas are not found. What organism is most likely the cause of this patient's acute illness?

- a. M. avium-intracellulare
- b. M. marinum
- c. M. leprae
- d. M. tuberculosis
- e. M. kansasii

7-43. A 41-year-old female is seen in the psychiatric clinic for a follow-up appointment. She has been taking an antidepressant for three weeks with some improvement in mood. However, she complains of drowsiness, palpitations, dry mouth, and feeling faint on standing. Which antidepressant is she taking?

- a. Amitriptyline
- b. Trazodone
- c. Fluoxetine
- d. Venlafaxine
- e. Bupropion

7-44. A 19-year-old female presents with urticaria that developed after she took aspirin for a headache. She has a history of chronic rhinitis, and physical examination reveals the presence of nasal polyps. This patient is at an increased risk of developing which one of the following pulmonary diseases following the ingestion of aspirin?

- a. Asthma
- b. Chronic bronchitis
- c. Emphysema
- d. Interstitial fibrosis
- e. Pulmonary hypertension

7-45. A 24-year-old female presents after having several "attacks" that last for about 24 hours. She states that during these "attacks" she develops nausea, vomiting, vertigo, and ringing in her ears. Physical examination reveals a sensorineural hearing loss. The pathology of her condition involves

- a. Acute suppurative inflammation
- b. Dilatation of the cochlear duct and saccule
- c. A cyst of the middle ear filled with keratin
- d. A tumor of the middle ear composed of lobules of cells in a highly vascular stroma
- e. New bone formation around the stapes and the oval window

7-46. A 58-year-old female presents as an outpatient with lethargy, fatigue, and cold intolerance. Thyroid function testing reveals a free T_4 level of 0.5 (0.7 to 2.0) and a TSH of 0.1 (0.5 to 5). The next best diagnostic test is

a. Thyroid scan and uptake
b. MRI of the pituitary
c. Prolactin
d. Thyroid autoantibodies
e. T_3

7-47. It is determined an infant suffers from Bruton's agammaglobulinemia. Which of the following pathogens will present the most serious threat to this child?

a. Measles virus
b. *Mycobacterium tuberculosis*
c. *Chlamydia trachomatis*
e. Varicella-zoster virus

7-48. A 25-year-old female in her 15th week of pregnancy presented with uterine bleeding and passage of a small amount of watery fluid and tissue. She is found to have a uterus that is much larger than estimated by her gestational dates. Her uterus is found to be filled with cystic, avascular, grapelike structures that do not penetrate the uterine wall. No fetal parts are found. The most likely diagnosis for this abnormality is

a. Partial hydatidiform mole
b. Complete hydatidiform mole
c. Invasive mole
d. Placental site trophoblastic tumor
e. Choriocarcinoma

7-49. A 4-year-old African male develops a rapidly enlarging mass that involves the right side of face. Biopsies of this lesion reveal a prominent "starry-sky" pattern produced by proliferating small, non-cleaved malignant lymphocytes. Based on this microscopic appearance, the diagnosis of Burkitt's lymphoma is made. This neoplasm most probably developed by which of the following mechanisms?

a. Gene amplification of erb-B
b. Point mutation of c-ras
c. Translocation of bcl-2 to the heavy chain region of chromosome 14
d. Translocation of c-abl to form the Philadelphia chromosome
e. Translocation of c-myc to the heavy chain region of chromosome 14

7-50. A 54-year-old male patient presents with a complaint of muscle weakness following exercise. Neurological examination reveals the muscles supplied by cranial nerves are most affected. You suspect myasthenia gravis. Your diagnosis is confirmed when lab tests indicate antibodies in the patient's blood against

a. Acetylcholinesterase
b. Muscle endplates
c. Cranial nerve synaptic membranes
d. Cranial nerve presynaptic membranes
e. Acetylcholine receptor

Answers

1-1. The answer is d. (*Cotran, 5/e, pp 649–651.*) Acute lymphoblastic leukemia (ALL) is primarily a disease of children and young adults that is characterized by the presence of numerous lymphoblasts within the bone marrow. These malignant cells may spill over into the blood and other organs. In contrast to myeloblasts, lymphoblasts do not contain myeloperoxidase, but they do stain positively with the PAS stain, acid phosphatase stain, and for the enzyme TdT. The French-American-British (FAB) classification of ALL divided ALL into three types based on the morphology of the proliferating lymphoblasts. L1 ALL, seen in about 85 percent of the cases of ALL, consists of small homogeneous blasts. L2 ALL, seen in only 15 percent of cases of ALL, but more common in adults, consists of lymphoblasts that are larger and more heterogeneous (pleomorphic) than L1 blasts. These cells also may contain nuclear clefts. The final type of FAB ALL is the L3 type, which is seen in less than 1 percent of the cases of ALL. This form is essentially the leukemic form of Burkitt's lymphoma. Like the malignant cells of Burkitt's lymphoma, these L3 ALL cells are large blasts with cytoplasmic vacuoles that stain positively with the oil-red-O lipid stain.

In contrast to the FAB classification of ALL, the immunologic classification of ALL is based on the developmental sequence of maturation of B lymphocytes and T lymphocytes. First it is necessary to determine whether the blasts have B cell or T cell markers. Most cases of ALL are of B cell origin; that is, the lymphoblasts express both CD19 and DR. A few cases of ALL are of T cell origin; the lymphoblasts lack CD19 and DR and instead express T cell antigens CD2, 5, and 7. Many patients with T-ALL have a mediastinal mass and are clinically similar to cases of lymphoblastic lymphoma. To subclassify B-ALL, first determine if surface immunoglobulin (sIg) is present. Mature B-ALL cells (L3 ALL or Burkitt's lymphoma) have surface immunoglobulin, which is not found in the other types of B-ALL. These mature cells typically lack TdT, which is a marker for more immature cells. Next determine if there is cytoplasmic μ present. Cytoplasmic μ chains are specific for pre-B ALL cells, which has a characteristic translocation t(1;19). Finally the B-cell ALL cells that lack both surface Ig and cytoplasmic μ are called early pre-B ALL and are separated into the CALLA (CD10) positive and CALLA negative types.

1-2. The answer is e. *(Murray, 5/e, pp 128–129.)* Since the boy received his booster within the last 2 years, his level of immunity should be adequate. If an individual has no history of immunization, both antitoxin (for temporary, fast protection) and toxoid (for future protection) should be given at different sites.

1-3. The answer is c. *(Kandel, 3/e, p 543.)* A CT scan of Helen's head was done in the emergency room, which showed a new infarct or stroke in the genu and anterior portion of the posterior limb of the left internal capsule. This is the region of the internal capsule through which most of the fibers of the corticospinal and corticobulbar tracts pass in a somatotopically organized fashion before entering the brainstem. Because most of these fibers pass through a very small region, a small infarct can cause deficits in a wide distribution of areas. In this case, Helen has weakness on her face and tongue, causing her slurred speech, in addition to weakness of her arm and leg. In addition, since somatosensory fibers destined for the postcentral gyrus occupy a position in the internal capsule caudal to the corticospinal tract fibers, these fibers are spared and Helen has no sensory deficits. The only other area in the central nervous system that can cause a pure motor hemiparesis is the basilar pons, an area through which corticospinal and corticobulbar fibers also run. The vascular supply of this region consists of perforators from the basilar artery, which are small and subject to atherosclerotic disease.

1-4. The answer is a. *(Kandel, 3/e, p 1042.)* The internal capsule is supplied primarily by the lenticulostriate branches of the middle cerebral artery. In addition, portions of the posterior limb of the internal capsule are supplied by the anterior choroidal artery, a branch of the internal carotid artery. Both the lateral striate branches and the anterior choroidal artery are small branches of larger arteries, and are more susceptible to damage (atherosclerosis) from high blood pressure and diabetes than the larger vessels.

I-5. The answer is c. *(Kandel, 3/e, p 543.)* The corticospinal and cortico-bulbar tracts contain motor fibers originating in the precentral gyrus, mediating voluntary motor function of the face, arms, legs, and trunk. They pass through the internal capsule to the crus cerebri in the midbrain. The spinothalamic tract is a sensory tract and could not cause the observed deficits. The rubrospinal tract only affects the spinal cord.

I-6. The answer is c. *(Wilson-Pauwels, p 86.)* Helen's forehead is unaffected by the lesion because the forehead is bilaterally represented on the cortex, so the right side retains innervation despite a lesion in the left internal capsule. Motor fibers from each side pass into the internal capsule ipsilaterally, so a lesion in the internal capsule will not affect the forehead. This type of finding is called a "central seventh nerve lesion," because it represents a lesion in the CNS superior to the level of the seventh nerve nucleus, where the fibers from both sides of the forehead coalesce.

I-7. The answer is d. *(Cotran, 5/e, pp 265, 459–461.)* Neuroblastomas are malignant tumors of the adrenal medulla that occur in very young patients who present with an abdominal mass. Histologically, these tumors are composed of small cells forming Homer-Wright rosettes, which are groups of cells arranged in a ring around a central mass of pink neural filaments. Electron microscopy reveals neurosecretory granules within the cytoplasm of the tumor cells, while immunohistochemical stains are positive for neuron-specific enolase (NSE). These highly aggressive tumors are unique because some will spontaneously regress and some will de-differentiate into benign tumors, such as ganglioneuromas. Three distinct chromosomal abnormalities are associated with neuroblastomas. These abnormalities include near-terminal deletion of part of the short arm of chromosome 1 (partial monosomy 1), homogeneously staining regions (HSR) of chromosome 2, and multiple double minute chromatin bodies. The latter two are the result of amplification of the oncogene *N-myc*. The number of *N-myc* copies correlates with the aggressiveness of the tumor. De-differentiation of a neuroblastoma into a benign ganglioneuroma is associated with a marked reduction in this gene amplification. In contrast, deletion of chromosome 11 is associated with nephroblastoma (Wilm's tumor), a malignant tumor of the kidney found in young patients. This chromosome abnormality is associated with deletion of WT-1, a tumor suppressor gene.

I-8. The answer is b. (*DiPalma, 4/e, pp 702–703. Hardman and Limbird, 9/e, p 1077.*) Unlike the other listed drugs, oxacillin is resistant to penicillinase. The other four agents are broad-spectrum penicillins, while oxacillin is generally specific for gram-positive microorganisms. Use of penicillinase-resistant penicillins should be reserved for infections caused by penicillinase-producing staphylococci.

I-9. The answer is c. (*Damjanov, 10/e, pp 1115–1116, 1325–1326. Cotran, 5/e, pp 1038–1039, 1063.*) Neisseria gonorrhoeae is a very common bacterium in this country that causes acute pelvic inflammatory disease with salpingitis as a result of venereal infection. Tuboovarian abscesses may develop from this bacterium, as well as other bacteria, but these organisms are susceptible to penicillin therapy. In the presence of unresponsiveness to penicillin, consideration should be given to Bacteroides species, which are important anaerobic gram-negative bacilli and are generally refractory to penicillin. These anaerobic bacteria may produce serious infections if uncontrolled. Chlamydiae, while considered to be nongonococcal in origin, are nevertheless important agents in venereal transmission and often are contracted at the same time as Neisseria species. When the gonococcus is adequately treated with penicillin, and symptoms continue, there may have been concurrent infection with chlamydia that is not responsive to penicillin but is sensitive to tetracycline. Adenoviruses are responsible for keratoconjunctivitis, tracheobronchitis, pneumonia in children, acute gastroenteritis, and occasionally hemorrhagic cystitis, but are not ordinarily causative in pelvic inflammatory disease.

I-10. The answer is e. (*Cotran, 5/e, pp 549, 555–556, 565–566.*) Plaques or vegetations are found in characteristic locations within the heart in several diseases. The carcinoid syndrome is characterized by episodic flushing, diarrhea, bronchospasm, and cyanosis. These symptoms are caused by the release of vasoactive amines, such as serotonin, from carcinoid tumors. These substances are inactivated by enzymes such as monoamine oxidase, which are found in the liver, lung, and brain. Therefore cardiac symptoms are found only in patients with liver metastases, which bypass the inactivation of the liver itself. The cardiac lesions are found on the right side of the heart since the active metabolites secreted by the tumor are inactivated in the lung and do not reach the left side of the heart. The cardiac lesions consist of fibrous plaques found on the tricuspid and pulmonic valves. In contrast, plaques in the left atrium are seen in chronic rheumatic heart disease and are called MacCallum's patches. Vegetations also occur in rheumatic heart disease; these are small and are found in a row along the lines of closure of the valve. Amyloid deposits may be found in the heart secondary to multiple myeloma, or as an isolated event, such as in senile cardiac amyloidosis. Grossly the walls of the heart may be thickened, and there may be multiple, small nodules on the left atrial endocardial surface. Iron overload can affect the heart as a result of hereditary hemochromatosis or hemosiderosis. Grossly the heart is a rust-brown color and resembles the heart in idiopathic dilated cardio-myopathy. In hypothyroidism the heart is characteristically flabby, enlarged, and dilated, which results in decreased cardiac output. This reduced circulation results in a characteristic symptom of hypothy-roidism, cold sensitivity. Histologically there is an interstitial muco-polysaccharide edema fluid within the heart.

1-11. The answer is b. (*McPhee, 2/e, p 552; Fauci, 14/e, pp 2092–2097.*) This patient has classic testosterone deficiency, as evidenced by the low sperm count and elevated gonadotropic hormones.

1-12. The answer is a. (*Cotran, 5/e, pp 283–284.*) Many chemicals are asso-ciated with an increased incidence of malignancy. These substances are called chemical carcinogens. Although there are direct acting chemical car-cinogens, such as the direct acting alkylating agents that are used in chemotherapy, most organic carcinogens first require conversion to a more reactive compound. Polycyclic aromatic hydrocarbons, aromatic amines, and azo dyes must be metabolized by cytochrome P450-dependent mixed function oxidases to active metabolites. Vinyl chloride is metabolized to an epoxide and is associated with angiosarcoma of the liver, not hepatocellular carcinoma. Azo dyes, such as butter yellow and scarlet red, are metabolized to active compounds that have induced hepatocellular cancer in rats, but no human cases have been reported. Beta-naphthylamine is an exception to the general rule involving cytochrome P450, as the hydrolysis of the nontoxic conjugate occurs in the urinary bladder by the urinary enzyme glu-curonidase. In the past there has been an increase in bladder cancer in work-ers in the aniline dye and rubber industries that have been exposed to these compounds. Aflatoxin B_1, a natural product of the fungus *Aspergillus flavus*, is metabolized to an epoxide. The fungus can grow on improperly stored peanuts and grains and is associated with the high incidence of hepatocellular carcinoma in some areas of Africa and the Far East. Hepatitis B virus is also highly associated with liver cancer in these regions.

1-13. The answer is a. (*Cotran, 5/e, pp 843–849. Chandrasoma, 3/e, pp 641–643.*) Several types of viruses are implicated as being causative agents of viral hepatitis. Each of these has unique characteristics. Hepatitis A virus, an RNA picornavirus, is transmitted through the fecal-oral route (including shellfish) and is called "infectious hepatitis." It is associated with small outbreaks of hepatitis in the United States, especially in young children at day care centers. Hepatitis B virus, which causes "serum hepatitis," is associated with the development of a serum sickness-like syndrome in about 10 percent of patients. Immune complexes of antibody and HBsAg are present in patients with vasculitis. Hepatitis C virus is characterized by episodic elevations in serum transaminases, and also by fatty change in liver biopsy specimens. Hepatitis D virus is distinct in that it is a defective virus and needs HBsAg to be infective. Finally, hepatitis E virus is characterized by its water-borne transmission. It is found in underdeveloped countries and has an unusually high mortality in pregnant females. It is important to remember that the liver may be infected by other viruses, such as yellow fever virus, Ebstein-Barr virus (EBV, the causative agent of infectious mononucleosis), CMV, and herpes virus. The latter is characterized histologically by intranuclear eosinophilic inclusions (Cowdry bodies) and nuclei that have a "ground-glass" appearance.

1-14. The answer is c. (*Cotran, 5/e, pp 328–329.*) In the approximate center of the photomicrograph is the classic, refractile, double-walled spherule of the deep fungus *Coccidioides immitis*, which is several times the diameter of the largest inflammatory cell nearby. Coccidioidomycosis is endemic in California, Arizona, New Mexico, and parts of Nevada, Utah, and Texas, where it resides in the arid soils and is contracted by direct inhalation of airborne dust. If inhaled, it produces a primary pulmonary infection that is usually benign and self-limiting in immunologically competent persons, often with several days of fever and upper respiratory flu-like symptoms. However, certain ethnic groups, such as some blacks, Asians, and Filipinos, are at risk of developing a potentially lethal disseminated form of the disease that can involve the central nervous system. If the large, double-walled spherule containing numerous endospores can be demonstrated outside the lungs (e.g., in a skin biopsy), this is evidence of dissemination. Antibodies of high titers are detectable by means of complement fixation studies in patients undergoing spontaneous recovery. Amphotericin B is usually reserved for treating high-risk and disseminated infection. The cultured mycelia of the organism on Sabouraud's agar present a hazard for laboratory workers.

I-15. The answer is b. (*Fauci, 14/e, p 1975.*) The serum level of prolactin correlates roughly with the size of the tumor. Prolactin levels greater than 300 µg/L are most likely associated with macroadenoma. Increases in prolactin due to medications are usually less than 100. Microadenomas usually do not exceed levels of 200 to 300.

I-16. The answer is d. (*Cotran, 5/e, pp 601–603.*) The autoimmune hemolytic anemias are important causes of acute anemia in a wide variety of clinical states and can be separated into two main types: those secondary to "warm" antibodies and those reactive at cold temperatures. Warm-antibody autoimmune hemolytic anemias react at 37°C in vitro, are composed of IgG, and do not fix complement. They are found in patients with malignant tumors, especially leukemia-lymphoma; with use of such drugs as alpha methyldopa; and in the autoimmune diseases, especially lupus erythematosus. Cold-antibody autoimmune hemolytic anemia reacts at 4 to 6°C, fixes complement, is of the IgM type, and is classically associated with mycoplasma pneumonitis (pleuropneumonia-like organisms). These antibodies are termed cold agglutinins and may reach extremely high titers and cause intravascular red cell agglutination.

I-17. The answer is a. (*Coe, pp 1042–1052. Cotran, 5/e, pp 1223–1225. Greenspan, 5/e, pp 308–311.*) Paget's disease is also known as osteitis deformans because of its deforming capabilities (e.g., skull or femoral head enlargement). In this disease the serum calcium is normal, but there is an increase in osteoclastic activity (osteolytic lesions and elevated 24-h urine hydroxyproline) and an increase in osteoblastic activity (elevated osteocalcin and alkaline phosphatase). Patients with Paget's disease exhibit a marked increase in osteoid, and the bone actually enlarges. The osteoid is never normally mineralized in this disease. In this patient, the bone scan shows significant uptake of labeled bisphosphonates, which are incorporated into newly formed osteoid during bone formation. Her proximal femur is enlarged and no longer fits properly into the acetabulum, which results in the hip pain.

1-18. The answer is d. (*Baum, 3/e, pp 220–221.*) Temporomandibular disorder (TMD) involves pain in the oral cavity and grinding of the teeth. It affects either the jaw and/or the muscles in the face, head, neck, and shoulders. Anxiety and depression are major causal links in promoting grinding of the teeth both during the day and at night. This action produces chronic pain even without the jaw moving or the teeth grinding. The physiological or neurological etiology is still not clear, but studies have estimated that between one-third and one-half of the general population suffers from TMD. Less than five percent of these sufferers seek medical attention. Emotional factors such as depression, anxiety, distress, and sensitivity to pain are particularly important in developing and maintaining the chronic pain. Psychosocial efforts to reduce the stress and depression show moderate success, as have dental and general pain clinics where patients are educated about the disorder and taught behavioral techniques to relax and reduce the pain, through biofeedback. Psychosocial therapy has also been successfully combined with selected antidepressants to help reduce TMD.

1-19. The answer is c. (*Cotran, 5/e, pp 978–979.*) A much rarer cause of hypertension is renal artery stenosis, which may occur secondary to either an atheromatous plaque at the orifice of the renal artery or fibromuscular dysplasia of the renal artery. The former is more common in elderly men, while the latter is more common in young women. The decrease in blood flow to the kidney with the renal artery obstruction (the Goldblatt kidney) causes hyperplasia of the juxtaglomerular apparatus and increased renin production. This will produce increased secretion of angiotensin and aldosterone, which will lead to retention of sodium and water and produce hypertension. Increased levels of aldosterone will also produce a hyperkalemic alkalosis. The kidney with the stenosis of the renal artery will become small and shrunken due to the effects of chronic ischemia, but the stenosis protects this kidney from the effects of the increased blood pressure. The other kidney, however, is not protected and may develop microscopic changes of benign nephrosclerosis (hyaline arteriolosclerosis).

1-20. The answer is e. (*Davis, 4/e, p 1018.*) Koplik's spots are pathognomonic for measles. The measles virus is a paramyxovirus. In industrialized countries, vaccination has reduced the importance of this childhood infection (although U.S. incidence increased in 1989 and 1990). In developing countries, however, measles is a major killer of young children. In America, most states now require proof of immunity before school enrollment, and this has reduced the incidence of disease.

I-21. The answer is c. *(Fauci, 14/e, p 1986.)* This patient presents with a high suspicion for Cushing's syndrome. The initial step in the evaluation should be an overnight dexamethasone suppression test. Failure to suppress would indicate a high likelihood of Cushing's syndrome. A random cortisol test is not sufficient to screen for Cushing's syndrome. An ACTH test by itself is not useful.

I-22. The answer is d. *(Kandel, 3/e, p 388.)* Norma's head CT showed an old stroke in her left ventral thalamus and no new lesions. A stroke involving the ventral posterolateral nucleus of the thalamus, especially several months after the stroke, can produce an entity called the syndrome of Dejerine-Roussy, or "thalamic pain syndrome." Although there is sensory loss on the contralateral side, there is pain or discomfort out of proportion to the stimulus on the affected side of the body. Emotional disturbance aggravates the response. Some patients describe the sensation as "knife-like" or "hot." As the deficit (numbness) resolves, the pain may lessen. This syndrome may also occur in lesions of the parietal white matter and is thought to occur as a result of an imbalance of afferent sensory impulses.

I-23. The answer is b. *(Kandel, 3/e, pp 363, 707.)* Sensation of the limbs and trunk are projected through the ventral posterior lateral nucleus of the thalamus to the somatosensory cortex. Sensory information from the face is carried through the trigeminal system to the ventral posterior medial nucleus, from which it is projected to the somatosensory cortex.

I-24. The answer is d. *(Kandel, 3/e, p 362.)* The spinothalamic tract is the only sensory pathway listed that mediates pain.

I-25. The answer is e. *(Kandel, 3/e, p 393.)* The periaqueductal gray is one area of many which produces analgesia when stimulated in both animals and in humans. It is an area with a high density of opiate receptors and opioidergic neurons, and is thought to represent a key area in gating pain.

1-26. The answer is b. (*Cotran, 5/e, pp 4–11.*) The first effect of the interruption of blood flow (ischemia) to cells is the decrease in ATP production by aerobic cellular processes. This results in decreased oxidative phosphorylation by mitochondria and an increase in anaerobic glycolysis, which decreases intracellular pH. Decreasing ATP levels also decreases the functioning of the energy-dependent sodium pump, which results in an increased cellular influx of sodium ions and an increased efflux of potassium. The resultant net gain of intracellular ions causes isosmotic water accumulation and hydropic cellular swelling. These changes are characteristic of reversible cellular injury, but they are reversible if blood flow and oxygen supply are restored.

With prolonged ischemia, however, certain cellular events occur that are not reversible, even with restoration of oxygen supply. These cellular changes are referred to as irreversible cellular injury. This type of injury is characterized by severe damage to mitochondria (vacuole formation), extensive damage to plasma membranes and nuclei, and rupture of lysosomes. Severe damage to mitochondria is characterized by the influx of calcium ions into the mitochondria and the subsequent formation of large, flocculent densities within the mitochondria. These flocculent densities are characteristically seen in irreversibly injured myocardial cells that undergo reperfusion soon after injury. Less severe changes in mitochondria, such as mitochondrial swelling, are seen with reversible injury.

1-27. The answer is d. (*Gelehrter, pp 159–189. Isselbacher, 13/e, pp 369–371. Jorde, pp 102–105. Thompson, 5/e, pp 230–246.*) The case described in the question represents one of the commoner chromosomal causes of reproductive failure, Turner mosaicism. Turner syndrome represents a pattern of anomalies, including short stature, heart defects, and infertility. Turner syndrome is often associated with a 45,X karyotype (monosomy X) in females, but mosaicism (i.e., two or more cell lines in the same individual with different karyotypes) is common. However, chimerism (i.e., two cell lines in an individual arising from different zygotes, such as fraternal twins who do not separate) is extremely rare. Trisomy refers to three copies of one chromosome; euploidy, to a normal chromosome number; and monoploidy, to one set of chromosomes (haploidy in humans).

1-28. The answer is d. (*April, 3/e, pp 383–384.*) The diffuse central abdominal pain in the patient presented is probably referred pain from the loop of small bowel incarcerated within the herniated peritoneal sac. Compression of the bowel results in compromise of the blood supply and subsequent ischemic necrosis. The visceral afferent fibers from the distal small bowel travel along the blood vessels to reach the superior mesenteric plexus and lesser splanchnic nerves, which they follow to the T10-T11 levels of the spinal cord. The pain, therefore, is referred to (appears as if originating from) the T10-T11 dermatomes, which supply the umbilical region. Because the gut develops as a midline structure, visceral pain tends to be centrally located regardless of the adult location of any particular region of the gut. As a result of dilation of the inguinal canal by the hernial sac, however, the patient also experiences localized somatic pain mediated by the iliohypogastric, ilioinguinal, and genitofemoral nerves.

I-29. The answer is c. *(Noback, 5/e, p 247. Nolte, 3/e, pp 182–185.)* In order for a lesion to produce both an ipsilateral gaze paralysis and contralateral hemiplegia, it must be situated in a location where fibers regulating both lateral gaze and movements of the contralateral limbs lie close to each other. The only such location is the ventrocaudal aspect of the pons, where fibers of cranial nerve VI descend toward the ventral surface of the brainstem and where corticospinal fibers are descending toward the spinal cord. The other regions listed in the question do not meet this condition.

I-30. The answer is c. *(Hardman and Limbird, 9/e, p 1179. Katzung, 7/e, p 781.)* Amphotericin B may alter kidney function by decreasing creatinine clearance; if this occurs, the dose must be reduced. It also commonly increases potassium (K) clearance, leading to hypokalemia, and causes anemia and neurologic symptoms. A liposomal preparation may reduce the incidence of renal and neurologic toxicity. Vancomycin is less likely to cause kidney damage; if it does, the damage is less severe.

I-31. The answer is a. *(Cotran, 5/e, pp 284–286, 1169–1170.)* Hereditary factors are important in the development of many types of cancers. They are particularly important in several inherited neoplasia syndromes. The autosomal recessive DNA-chromosomal instability syndromes include ataxia-telan-giectasia, Bloom syndrome, Fanconi's anemia, and xeroderma pigmentosa. These disorders have in common abnormalities involving the normal repair of DNA. Patients with xeroderma pigmentosa have defective endo-nuclease activity, which normally repairs the pyrimidine dimers found in ultraviolet (UV) light damaged DNA. These patients have an increased incidence of skin cancers, including basal cell carcinoma, squamous cell carcinoma, and malignant melanoma. Wiskott-Aldrich syndrome, characterized by thrombocytopenia and eczema, is an immunodeficiency disease associated with an increased incidence of lymphomas and acute leukemias. Familial polyposis is characterized by the formation of numerous neoplastic adenomatous colon polyps. These individuals have a 100 percent risk of developing colorectal carcinoma unless surgery is performed. Sturge-Weber syndrome is a rare congenital disorder associated with venous angiomatous masses in the leptomeninges and ipsilateral port-wine nevi of the face. Multiple endocrine neoplasia (MEN) syndrome type I, Wermer syndrome, refers to the combination of adenomas of the pituitary, adenomas or hyperplasia of the parathyroid glands, and islet cell tumors of the pancreas.

1-32. The answer is e. *(Murray, 24/e, pp 377–378, 382–384. Stryer 4/e, pp 745–748.)* Orotic aciduria is the buildup of orotic acid due to a deficiency in one or both of the enzymes that convert it to UMP. Either orotate phosphoribosyltransferase and orotidylate decarboxylase are both defective, or the decarboxylase alone is defective. UMP is the precursor of UTP, CTP, and TMP. All of these end products normally act in some way to feedback inhibit the initial reactions of pyrimidine synthesis. Specifically, the lack of CTP inhibition allows aspartate transcarbamoylase to remain highly active and ultimately results in a buildup of orotic acid and the resultant orotic aciduria. The lack of CTP, TMP, and UTP leads to a decreased erythrocyte formation and megaloblastic anemia. Uridine treatment is effective since it can easily be converted to UMP by omnipresent tissue kinases and allow UPT, CTP, and TMP to be synthesized and feedback inhibit further orotic acid production.

1-33. The answer is c. *(Fauci, 14/e, p 603.)* LDH is an important marker to follow in any germ cell tumor. AFP elevation is seen only in nonseminoma, whereas β-hCG is seen in both nonseminoma and seminoma. The half-life of AFP is 5 to 7 days.

1-34. The answer is b. *(Cotran, 5/e, pp 133–135, 499–504, 936, 1312–1313.)* Dissecting aneurysms are usually the result of cystic medial necrosis of the aorta. This abnormality results from loss of elastic tissue in the media and is associated with hypertension and Marfan's syndrome. Most cases of dissecting aneurysms have a transverse tear in the intima and are located in the ascending aorta, just above the aortic ring. The pain caused by a dissecting aneurysm is similar to the pain caused by a myocardial infarction, but it extends into the abdomen as the dissection progresses. Additionally, the blood pressure is not decreased with a dissecting aneurysm unless the aorta itself has ruptured.

Berry aneurysms, found at the bifurcation of arteries in the circle of Willis, are due to congenital defects in the vascular wall. Rupture of these aneurysms may produce a fatal subarachnoid hemorrhage. Berry aneurysms have been noted in about one-sixth of patients with adult polycystic renal disease and account for death in about 10 percent of patients with this type of polycystic renal disease. Syphilitic (luetic) aneurysms occur in the thoracic aorta and may lead to luetic heart disease by producing insufficiency of the aortic valve. Mycotic (infectious) aneurysms result from microbial infection during septicemia, usually secondary to bacterial endocarditis. They are prone to rupture and hemorrhage. Ehlers-Danlos syndromes (EDSs) are a group of eight syndromes characterized by defects in collagen synthesis. In EDS IV there is deficient synthesis of type III collagen and a tendency to rupture of muscular arteries, including dissecting aneurysms of the aorta.

I-35. The answer is c. (*Cotran, 5/e, pp 682–694.*) Chronic obstructive pulmonary disease (COPD) is a term that refers to a group of disorders characterized by dyspnea and airway obstruction. The spectrum of COPD includes all the diseases listed in the question. Patients with bronchiectasis have a persistent, productive cough due to abnormally dilated bronchi, which are the result of a chronic necrotizing infection. Patients with Kartagener's syndrome have the triad of bronchiectasis, recurrent sinusitis, and situs inversus. This syndrome is caused by abnormal motility of the cilia, which is due to abnormalities of the dynein arms. Males with this condition tend to be sterile because of the ineffective motility of the tail of the sperm. Patients with asthma suffer from episodic wheezing due to bronchial smooth muscle hyperplasia and excess production of mucus. Extrinsic (allergic) asthma may be related to IgE (type I) immune reactions; intrinsic (nonallergic) asthma may be triggered by infections or drugs. Clinically there is an elevated eosinophil count in the peripheral blood, and Curschmann's spirals and Charcot-Leyden crystals may be found in the sputum. Chronic bronchitis is characterized by a productive cough that is present for at least 3 months in at least 2 consecutive years. There is hyper-plasia of mucous glands with hypersecretion due in large part to tobacco smoke. Emphysema is abnormal dilation of the alveoli due to destruction of the alveolar walls. Bronchiolitis is inflammation and scarring of bronchi-oles due mainly to tobacco smoke and air pollutants.

I-36. The answer is c. (*Hardman and Limbird, 9/e, pp 887, 889.*) Bile acid-binding resins bind more than just bile acids, and binding of simvastatin to cholestyramine is the most likely mechanism for decreased GI absorption. Cholestyramine may also bind to several other drugs, including digitalis, benzothiadiazides (thiazides), warfarin, vancomycin, thyroxine (T_4), and aspirin. Medications should be given one hour before or four hours after cholestyramine.

I-37. The answer is d. (*Moore, Embryology, 5/e, pp 15–18. Sadler, 7/e, pp 16–20.*) Spermatogenesis, the process by which spermatogonia undergo mitotic division to produce primary spermatocytes, occurs at 1°C (2°F) below normal body temperature. Subsequent meiotic divisions produce secondary spermatocytes with a bivalent haploid chromosome number and then sper-matids with a monovalent haploid chromosome number. The maturation of the spermatid, spermiogenesis, results in spermatozoa. Morphologically adult spermatozoa are moved to the epididymis where they become fully motile. In man the time period required for the progression from sper-matogonium to motile spermatozoon is 61 to 64 days.

I-38. The answer is b. (*Fauci, 14/e, p 1982.*) The best screening test for suspected acromegaly is a test for IGF-1. Random growth hormone varies too much to be useful. TSH and prolactin may be abnormal but are not diagnostic of acromegaly. Fasting blood sugar may be elevated in this patient, but again it is not diagnostic.

I-39. The answer is b. (*Adams, 6/e, pp 443–445, 453–459.*) This case is an example of a lesion of the left (usually dominant) parietal lobe, most often in the angular gyrus, with some involvement of the precentral gyrus in the posterior frontal lobe. There is contralateral upper motor neuron weakness (with a positive Babinski sign), as well as several cortical sensory defects, specifically, right-left confusion, agraphia (inability to write, independent of motor weakness), acalculia (inability to calculate), and finger agnosia (inability to designate the fingers). The latter four elements are sometimes referred to as Gerstmann syndrome by neurologists, and all represent spatial discriminatory functions of the parietal lobe (often the dominant parietal lobe, which is usually the left). The parietal lobe also subserves other visual-spatial functions such as construction of complex drawings. There are other locations within the central nervous system where upper motor neuron weakness can occur; however, the combination with parietal lobe signs can only occur in this location. If the damage was slightly more extensive, it may have involved Broca's area, causing aphasia.

I-40. The answer is d. (*Kandel, 3/e, pp 1041–1043.*) The artery serving this region (both posterior frontal and parietal lobes) is the right middle cerebral artery, which originates at the Circle of Willis. Because it continues in a nearly straight line from the internal carotid artery, it is a common route for small emboli formed from blood clots in the internal carotid artery. The bruit noted over the right common carotid artery in this patient is most likely a result of a thrombus (clot) which occludes part of the lumen of the artery. These emboli can occlude the middle cerebral artery because it is considerably smaller than the internal carotid artery. Since the middle cerebral artery has many branches through which an embolus may travel, but the territory of this stroke is large, it is likely that the embolus lodged in a more proximal location in this case.

I-41. The answer is b. (*Kandel, 3/e, pp 1043–1045.*) Morris's leg weakness includes a positive Babinski sign, which is an upper motor neuron sign. Although this type of weakness may occur in several locations in the central nervous system, the combination with the cortical parietal signs can only occur in the left precentral gyrus if there is to be one lesion.

I-42. The answer is a. (*Adams, 6/e, pp 443–445, 453–459.*) These deficits are visual-spatial in nature and are characteristic of damage to the dominant parietal lobe.

I-43. The answer is c. (*Cotran, 5/e, pp 138–144.*) One group of lysosomal storage diseases is characterized by the abnormal accumulation of sphingolipids (SL). Some types of sphingolipids are typically found within the central nervous system, and therefore abnormal accumulation of these substances will produce neurologic signs and symptoms. For example, ganglion cells within the retina, particularly at the periphery of the macula, may become swollen with excess sphingolipids. The affected area of the retina will appear pale when viewed through an ophthalmoscope. In contrast the normal color of the macula, which does not have accumulated substances, appears more red than normal. This is referred to as a cherry-red spot or a cherry-red macula. Substances that may produce this cherry-red spot include sphingomyelin, which is increased in individuals with Neiman-Pick's disease, and gangliosides, which may be increased in individuals with Tay-Sachs disease, Sandhoff's disease, or GM_1 gangliosidosis.

Autosomal recessive disorders tend to be more common in areas in which in-breeding is more common. An example of this is the increased frequency of several autosomal recessive genes in Ashkenazi Jews. "Ashkenazi" denotes an ethnic group, mostly of the Jewish faith, from Eastern Europe. People of this faith tend to marry other members of the faith. Two storage diseases that have a higher incidence in Ashkenazi Jews are Tay-Sachs disease and Type I Gaucher disease. Tay-Sachs disease is due to a deficiency of hexosaminidase A. This same enzyme is decreased in patients with Sandhoff's disease. Hexosaminidase A is composed of an α subunit and a β subunit. In contrast, hexosaminidase B is composed of two β subunits. Patients with Tay-Sachs disease have a deficiency of the α subunit. Therefore, they have a deficiency of hexosaminidase A but not hexosaminidase B. In contrast, patients with Sandhoff's disease have a deficiency of the β subunit, and they have a deficiency of both hexosaminidase A and hexosaminidase B. In patients with Tay-Sachs disease, accumulation of GM_2 ganglioside occurs within many tissues including the heart, liver, spleen, and brain. Electron microscopy reveals cytoplasmic whorled lamellar bodies within lysosomes. There are several clinical forms of Tay-Sachs disease, but the most severe is the infantile type. Patients develop mental retardation, seizures, motor incoordination, blindness (amaurosis), and usually die by the age of three.

Type I Gaucher's disease is due to a deficiency of β-glucocerebrosidase. Patients may have increased serum levels of acid phosphatase, an enzyme that is typically found in the prostate, erythrocytes, and platelets. Patients with Gaucher's disease have excess glucocerebrosides accumulation within phagocytic cells, not ganglion cells. Sphingomyelinase is decreased in patients with Neiman-Picks disease, while aryl-sulfatase is decreased in patients with metachromatic leukodystrophy (MLD).

1-44. The answer is a. _(Baum, 3/e, pp 297–301.)_ Progressive muscle relaxation, or a reasonable variation, can serve as a powerful therapeutic technique for treating generalized anxiety, insomnia, headaches, neck tension, and mild forms of agitated depression. It has also effectively been used to reduce pain, the side effects of cancer chemotherapy, nausea, and mild hypertension, preferably before pharmacological intervention. Relaxation therapy is based on the premise and observation that muscle tension is a physiological response to anxiety and stress. There is a significant reduction in experienced anxiety if tense muscles can be relaxed. Muscle relaxation also can change the physiological activation process. The Jacobson relaxation procedure involves tensing selected muscles for about ten seconds, and then completely relaxing them and noticing the difference in sensation. Eventually, the patient is able to relax particular muscle groups from their present level of tension. Other effective methods of relaxation include systematic deep breathing, transcendental meditation, and Yoga.

1-45. The answer is b. _(Cotran, 5/e, pp 1124–1125, 1131–1133.)_ The consequences of excess or inadequate thyroid hormone are directly attributed to abnormalities involving the normal functioning of thyroid hormones, such as regulation of body processes. For example, excess thyroid hormone (hyperthyroidism) results in weight loss (increased lipolysis) despite increased food intake, heat intolerance, increased heart rate, tremor, nervousness, and weakness (due to loss in muscle mass). Inadequate levels of thyroid hormone (hypothyroidism) produce different signs and symptoms in children compared to older children and adults. In young children hypothyroidism produces cretinism, a disease that is characterized by marked retardation of physical and mental growth (severe mental retardation). Patients develop dry, rough skin and a protuberant abdomen. Characteristic facial features include periorbital edema, a flattened broad nose, and a large, protuberant tongue. In contrast, hypothyroidism in older children and adults produces myxedema. This disease is characterized by a decrease in the metabolic rate, which can result in multiple different signs and symptoms, such as cold intolerance and weight gain. Neurologic features of this abnormality include slowing of intellectual and motor function (fatigue, lethargy, and slow speech), apathy, sleepiness, depression, paranoia, and prolonged relaxation phase in deep tendon reflexes ("hung-up" reflexes). Other signs and symptoms of hypothyroidism include dry skin and brittle hair, which can produce hair loss; decreased erythropoiesis,

which produces a normochromic normocytic anemia; increased cholesterol, which increases the risk of atherosclerosis; and myxedema, which is
the increased interstitial deposition of mucopolysaccharides. The latter
abnormality can result in diffuse non-pitting edema of the skin, hoarseness,
and enlargement of the heart. Other systems affected by hypothyroidism
include the heart, the GI tract, and the GU tract. Patients may develop a
slowed heart rate and decrease stroke volume (resulting in cool, pale skin),
constipation, and impotence in men, and menorrhagia and anovulatory
cycles in women.

Graves' disease (diffuse toxic hyperplasia) is an autoimmune disorder
that clinically produces hyperthyroidism. Other common causes of primary
diseases of the thyroid that cause hyperthyroidism include toxic multinodular goiter and toxic adenoma. These three diseases have in common
the word "toxic," which refers to the symptoms of hyperthyroidism. Goi-
ters and adenomas are not necessarily "toxic," and these patients may
instead be euthyroid, e.g., diffuse nontoxic (simple) goiter, multinodular
nontoxic goiter, and nontoxic adenoma. Uncommon causes of hyperthyroidism include choriocarcinomas, hydatidiform moles (both of which
may produce TSH-like substances in addition to chorionic gonadotropins), struma ovarii (a monodermal teratoma of the ovary that is composed
of thyroid), and TSH-secreting pituitary tumors.

1-46. The answer is c. (*Damjanov, 10/e, pp 886–887, 928–930. Duchin,
N Engl J Med 330: 949–955, 1994.*) The Hantavirus genus belongs to the
Bunyaviridae family and includes the causative agent of a group of diseases
that occur throughout Europe and Asia and are referred to as hemorrhagic
fever with renal syndrome. The characteristic features of this syndrome are
hematologic abnormalities, renal involvement, and increased vascular permeability. Respiratory involvement is generally minimal in these diseases.
Although several species of rodents in the United States were known to be
infected with Hantavirus, no human cases had been reported until an out-
break of severe, often fatal respiratory illness occurred in the United States
in May 1993 in the Four Corners area of New Mexico, Arizona, Colorado,
and Utah. This illness resulted from a new member of the genus Hantavirus
that caused a severe disease characterized by a prodromal fever, myalgia,
pulmonary edema, and hypotension. The main distinguishing feature of
this illness, which is called Hantavirus pulmonary syndrome, is noncardio-
genic pulmonary edema resulting from increased permeability of the

pulmonary capillaries. Laboratory features common to both Hantavirus pulmonary syndrome and hemorrhagic fever with renal syndrome include leukocytosis, atypical lymphocytes, thrombocytopenia, coagulopathy, and decreased serum protein concentrations. Abdominal pain, which can mimic an acute abdomen, may be found in both Hantavirus pulmonary syndrome and hemorrhagic fever with renal syndrome.

Dengue fever virus is a type of flavivirus, which are similar to alphaviruses. Dengue fever (breakbone fever) is initially similar to influenza but then progresses to a rash, muscle pain, joint pain, and bone pain. It can produce a potentially fatal hemorrhagic disorder. Yellow fever virus is another flavivirus that causes yellow fever. It is spread by a mosquito and produces characteristic coagulative necrosis of liver acinar zone 2 (midzonal necrosis). The necrotic hepatocytes, produced by the process of apoptosis in the absence of inflammation, result in Councilman bodies. Because of liver failure, patients become jaundiced (yellow fever) and may vomit clotted blood ("black vomit"). Another flavivirus is the cause of St. Louis encephalitis, which is spread by the Culex mosquito. Alphavirus, a type of togavirus, is similar to flaviviruses. They are the prototypical arboviruses, which are arthropod-born viruses. Clinical diseases include EEE (eastern equine encephalitis), WEE (western equine encephalitis), and VEE (Venezuelan equine encephalitis). Ebola virus is a Filoviridae that causes a severe hemorrhagic fever. Outbreaks occur in Africa and typically make the national news.

I-47. The answer is a. (*Hardman and Limbird, 9/e, p 444.*) This patient has the serotonin syndrome. Serotonin is already present in increased amounts in synapses because of blockade of its reuptake by the selective serotonin reuptake inhibitors (SSRI). The amount of serotonin present is further increased when breakdown by MAO is inhibited. The serotonin syndrome can be life threatening.

I-48. The answer is c. (*Levinson, Jawetz, 4/e, pp 113–114.*) The symptoms of Legionnaires' disease are similar to those of mycoplasmal pneumonia and influenza. Affected persons are moderately febrile, complain of pleuritic chest pain, and have a dry cough. Unlike *Klebsiella* and *Staphylococcus*, *Legionella pneumophila* exhibits fastidious growth requirements. Charcoal yeast extract agar either with or without antibiotics is the preferred isolation medium. While sputum may not be the specimen of choice for *Legionella*, the discovery of small Gram negative rods by direct fluorescent antibody (FA) technique should certainly heighten suspicion of the disease. *L. pneumophila* is a facultative intracellular pathogen and enters macrophages without activating their oxidizing capabilities. The organisms bind to macrophage C receptors, which promote engulfment.

1-49. The answer is b. (*Cotran, 5/e, pp 757–758.*) Achalasia, which means "unrelaxed," is a term that describes the absence of normal lower esophageal sphincter (LES) relaxation. This disease results from decreased or absent ganglion cells in the myenteric plexus in the body of the esophagus. The etiology of this neuronal loss is unknown in many cases; however, some cases are secondary to other diseases, such as diabetes mellitus, amyloidosis, sarcoidosis, and Chagas disease, which is caused by *Trypanosoma cruzi*. Because of the increased LES pressure and the absence of peristaltic waves in the lower esophagus, the esophagus in these patients is dilated and tortuous above the level of the LES. Barium x-ray studies reveal this dilated esophagus. The distal esophagus has a characteristic "beak-like" appearance. Patients with achalasia have an increased risk of developing aspiration pneumonia and squamous cell carcinoma.

1-50. The answer is e. (*McPhee, 2/e, p 529; Barron, 2/e, pp 241–244.*) Factors I, VII, VIII, IX, X, and XII are increased in pregnancy. Factors II, III, IV, V, VI, XI, and XIII are unchanged.

BLOCK 2

Answers

2-1. The answer is a. (*Hardman and Limbird, 9/e, p 338. Katzung, 7/e, p 427.*) Ester-type local anesthetics are mainly hydrolyzed by pseudocholinesterases. Amide-type local anesthetics are hydrolyzed by microsomal enzymes in the liver. Of the listed agents, only lidocaine is an amide and can be influenced by liver dysfunction.

2-2. The answer is b. (*Cotran, 5/e, pp 1159, 1169–1170. Rubin, 2/e, pp 1132, 1140.*) Combinations of neoplasms affecting different endocrine organs in the same patient are referred to as multiple endocrine neoplasia (MEN) syndromes. There are several types of MEN syndromes. Patients with type I MEN syndrome (Wermer syndrome) have pituitary adenomas, parathyroid hyperplasia (or adenomas), and neoplasms of the pancreatic islets. The latter most commonly are gastrinomas, which secrete gastrin and produce the Zollinger-Ellison syndrome. Type IIa MEN syndrome (Sipple syndrome) is characterized by the combination of medullary carcinoma of the thyroid, pheochromocytoma of the adrenal medulla, and hyperparathyroidism. MEN type IIb syndrome (also known as type III) is associated with medullary carcinoma of the thyroid, pheochromocytoma of the adrenal medulla, and multiple mucocutaneous neuromas.

In contrast to the MEN syndromes, combinations of autoimmune diseases affecting different endocrine organs is called polyglandular syndromes. There are several types of polyglandular syndromes. Patients with type I polyglandular autoimmune syndrome have at least two of the triad of Addison's disease, hypoparathyroidism, and mucocutaneous candidiasis. Type II polyglandular syndrome (Schmidt's syndrome) is not associated with either hypoparathyroidism or mucocutaneous candidiasis, but instead is associated with autoimmune thyroid disease (Hashimoto's thyroiditis) and insulin-dependent diabetes mellitus.

2-3. The answer is c. (*Joklik, 20/e, pp 1060–1063. Rubin, 2/e, pp 341–344.*) Human parvovirus may cause a serious aplastic crisis in patients with an underlying chronic hemolytic anemia. In children, infection with parvovirus produces a characteristic rash, called erythema infectiosum or fifth disease, which first appears on the face and is described as a "slapped cheek" appearance. Human parvovirus infection in adults produces a nonspecific syndrome of fever, malaise, headache, myalgia, vomiting, and a transient rash. Arthralgia is more common in adults than in children. There are many types of rhinoviruses, which are causative agents of the common cold (coryza). This infection is characterized by rhinorrhea, pharyngitis, cough, and a low-grade fever. Parainfluenza viruses, single-stranded RNA viruses that kill ciliated respiratory epithelial cells, are the most common cause of croup, which is a disease of children characterized by a barking sound on inspiration. Rubeola virus, an RNA virus, is the cause of measles. After an incubation of 10 to 21 days, measles is characterized by fever, rhinorrhea, cough, skin lesions, and mucosal lesions (Koplik spots). Rubella virus, another RNA virus, produces a mild, acute febrile illness, but if the infection occurs in the first trimester of pregnancy it can produce developmental abnormalities such as cardiac lesions, ocular abnormalities, deafness, and mental retardation.

2-4. The answer is d. (*Jawetz, 19/e, pp 461–462.*) In a small number of patients with acute hepatitis B infection, HBsAg can never be detected. In others, HBsAg becomes negative before the onset of the disease or before the end of the clinical illness. In such patients with acute hepatitis, hepatitis B virus infection may only be established by the presence of anti-hepatitis B core IgM (anti-HBc IgM), a rising titer of anti-HBc, or the subsequent appearance of anti-HBsAg.

2-5. The answer is b. (*Cotran, 5/e, pp 666–667. Rubin, 2/e, pp 1034–1036.*) Langerhans cell histiocytosis, previously known as histiocytosis X, refers to a spectrum of clinical diseases that are associated with the proliferation of Langerhans cells. These cells, not to be confused with the Langhans-type giant cells found in caseating granulomas of tuberculosis, have Fc receptors, HLA-D/DR antigens, and react with CD1 antibodies. These cells have distinctive granules seen by electron microscopy that are rod-shaped organelles resembling tennis rackets. They are called LC (Langerhans cells) granules, pentilaminar bodies, or Birbeck granules. There are three general clinical forms of Langerhans cell histiocytosis. Acute disseminated Langerhans cell histiocytosis (Letterer-Siwe disease) affects children before the age of three. These children have cutaneous lesions that resemble seborrhea, hepatosplenomegaly, and lymphadenopathy.

The Langerhans cells infiltrate the marrow, which leads to anemia, thrombocytopenia, and recurrent infections. The clinical course is usually rapidly fatal; however, with intensive chemotherapy 50 percent of patients may survive 5 years. Multifocal Langerhans cell histiocytosis (Hand-Schuller-Christian disease) usually begins between the second and sixth year of life. The characteristic triad consists of bone lesions, particularly in the calvarium and the base of the skull, diabetes insipidus, and exophthalmos. These lesions are the result of proliferations of Langerhans cells. Lesions around the hypothalamus lead to decreased ADH production and signs of diabetes insipidus. Unifocal Langerhans cell histiocytosis (eosinophilic granuloma), seen in older patients, is usually a unifocal disease, most often affecting the skeletal system. The lesions are granulomas that contain a mixture of lipid-laden Langerhans cells, macrophages, lymphocytes, and eosinophils.

Sarcoidosis is characterized by a proliferation of activated macrophages that form granulomas. It is not a proliferation of Langerhans cells. Dermatopathic lymphadenitis refers to a chronic lymphadenitis that affects the lymph nodes draining the sites of chronic dermatologic diseases. The lymph nodes have hyperplasia of the germinal follicles and accumulation of melanin and hemosiderin pigment by the phagocytic cells.

2-6. The answer is c. *(Wilson-Pauwels, p 47.)* Damage to the trochlear nerve causes weakness of the superior oblique muscle, resulting in the inability of the orbit to deviate downward when the eye is intorted. In order to compensate for the classically vertical double vision, the patient tends to tilt his head to the contralateral side, causing the contralateral eye to intort.

2-7. The answer is d. *(Wilson-Pauwels, pp 45–47.)* The trochlear nerve supplies the superior oblique muscle.

2-8. The answer is b. *(Wilson-Pauwels, pp 43–44.)* The trochlear nerve is the only nerve to decussate peripherally and, also, to emerge from the dorsal aspect of the brainstem. In this case, the damaged nerve emerged from the right (contralateral) dorsal midbrain.

2-9. The answer is d. *(Wilson-Pauwels, p 46.)* The action of the superior oblique muscle is to rotate the eye medially and downward.

2-10. The answer is d. (*Cotran, 5/e, pp 25–26, 859. Chandrasoma, 3/e, pp 8–10.*) Free fatty acids are normally taken up by the liver and esterified to triglyceride, converted to cholesterol, oxidized into ketone bodies, or incorporated into phospholipids that can be excreted as very low density lipoproteins (VLDL). Abnormalities involving these normal metabolic pathways may lead to the accumulation of triglyceride within the hepatocytes. This accumulation of triglyceride is called fatty change or steatosis. Examples of abnormalities that produce hepatic steatosis include diseases that cause excess delivery of free fatty acids to the liver or diseases that cause impaired lipoprotein synthesis. Excess delivery of free fatty acids occurs in conditions that increase mobilization of adipose tissue, such as starvation, corticosteroid use, and diabetes mellitus. Impaired lipoprotein synthesis occurs with carbon tetrachloride poisoning, phosphorous poisoning, and protein malnutrition.

Alcohol can produce hepatic steatosis by several mechanisms, such as increased fatty acid synthesis, decreased triglyceride utilization, decreased fatty acid oxidation, decreased lipoprotein excretion, and increased lipolysis. Ethanol is taken up by the liver and is converted into acetaldehyde by either alcohol dehydrogenase (the major pathway), microsomal P-450 oxidase, or peroxisomal catalase. These pathways also convert NAD (nicotinamide adenine dinucleotide) to NADH. This excess production of NADH changes the normal hepatic metabolism away from catabolism of fats and toward anabolism of fats (lipid synthesis). This results in decreased mitochondrial oxidation of fatty acids and increased hepatic production of triglyceride. Ethanol also increases lipolysis and inhibits the release of lipoproteins. Increased lipolysis increases the amount of free fatty acids that reach the liver.

2-11. The answer is c. (*Cotran, 5/e, pp 1033–1034. Larsen, 1/e, pp 247–253.*) The paired genital ducts consist of the mesonephric (Wolffian) duct, which extends from the mesonephros to the cloaca, and the paramesonephric (Müllerian) duct, which runs parallel and lateral to the wolffian duct. The mesonephric ducts in males, if stimulated by testosterone secreted by the Leydig cells, develop into the vas deferens, epididymis, and seminal vesicles. In contrast because normal females do not secrete testosterone, the wolffian ducts regress and form vestigial structures. They may, however, form mesonephric cysts in the cervix or vulva, or they may form Gartner duct cysts in the vagina. The cranial group of mesonephric tubules, the epoöphoron, remain as vestige structures in the broad ligament above the ovary, while the caudal group of mesonephric tubules, the paroöphoron, form vestigial structures in the broad ligament beside the ovary. The paramesonephric (Müllerian) ducts in the female form the fallopian tubes, the uterus, the uppermost vaginal wall, and the hydatid of Morgagni. The lower portion of the vagina and the vestibule develop from the urogenital sinus. Males secrete Müllerian inhibiting factor (MIF) from the Sertoli cells of the testes, which causes regression of the Müllerian ducts. This results in the formation of the vestigial appendix testis. The metanephric duct in both sexes will form the ureter, renal pelvis, calyces, and renal collecting tubules. Several abnormalities result from abnormal embryonic development of the Müllerian ducts. Uterine agenesis may result from abnormal development of fusion of these paired paramesonephric ducts. Developmental failure of the inferior portions of the Müllerian ducts results in a double uterus, while failure of the superior portions to fuse (incomplete fusion) may form a bicornuate uterus. Retarded growth of one of the paramesonephric ducts along with incomplete fusion to the other paramesonephric ducts will result in the formation of a bicornuate uterus with a rudimentary horn.

2-12. The answer is b. (*Cotran, 5/e, pp 557–562.*) The cardiomyopathies (CMP) may be classified into primary and secondary forms. The primary forms are mainly idiopathic (unknown cause). Most of these secondary cardiomyopathies result in a dilated cardiomyopathy that is characterized by congestion and four chamber dilation with hypertrophy. The walls are either of normal thickness or they may be thinner than normal. This results in a flabby, globular, banana-shaped heart that is hypocontracting. The microscopic appearance is not distinctive. The ventricles may have mural thrombi. The causes of secondary dilated CMP are many and include alcoholism (the most common cause in the United States), metabolic disorders, and toxins. Examples of the latter include cobalt, which has been used in beer as a foam stabilizer, anthracyclines, cocaine, and iron, the deposition of which is seen in patients with hemochromatosis. The anthracycline Adriamycin, which is used in chemotherapy, causes lipid peroxidation of myofiber membranes. One final form of DCM develops in the last trimester of pregnancy or the first six months after delivery. About 1/2 of these patients recover full cardiac function.

Other forms of cardiomyopathies include a hypertrophic form, a restrictive form, and an obliterative form. In hypertrophic CMP the major gross abnormality is within the interventricular septum, which is usually thicker than the left ventricle. Constrictive (restrictive) CMP is associated with amyloidosis, sarcoidosis, endomyocardial disease, or storage diseases. These abnormalities produce a stiff, hypocontracting heart.

2-13. The answer is d. (*Cotran, 5/e, pp 1298–1300. Rubin, 2/e, p 1439.*) The clinical constellation of altered sensorium and papilledema should call to mind the presence of intracranial pressure, regardless of the cause, which can be due to cerebral edema, tumor mass, or, more commonly, intracranial bleeding with hematoma formation. If the pressure is severe enough, downward displacement of the cerebellar tonsils into the foramen magnum may occur, producing further compression on the brainstem with consequent hemorrhage into the pons and midbrain (Duret hemorrhages). This is nearly always associated with death, since the vital centers, including respiratory control, are located in these regions. Subdural as well as epidural hemorrhages are sufficient to cause critical downward displacement of the cerebellar tonsils. The situation can be remedied with appropriate neurosurgical intervention. In this situation, the downward displacement could be due to hemorrhage-hematoma formation into the posterior intracranial fossa, caused by either a direct (coup) or an indirect (contrecoup) blow to the occiput.

2-14. The answer is e. (*Cotran, 5/e, pp 114–116, 1014–1015.*) Infarcts are localized areas of ischemic coagulative necrosis. They can be classified on the basis of their color into either red or white infarcts, or by the presence or absence of bacterial contamination into either septic or bland infarcts. White infarcts, also referred to as pale or anemic infarcts, are usually the result of arterial occlusion. They are found in solid organs such as the heart, spleen, and kidneys. Red or hemorrhagic infarcts, in contrast, may result from either arterial or venous occlusion. They occur in organs with a dual blood supply, such as the lung, or in organs with extensive collateral circulation, such as the small intestine and brain. These infarcts are hemorrhagic because there is bleeding into the necrotic area from the adjacent arteries and veins which remain patent. Hemorrhagic infarcts also occur in organs in which the venous outflow is obstructed, that is venous occlusion. Examples of this include torsion of the ovary or testis. In the latter twisting of the spermatic cord occludes the venous outflow, but the arterial inflow remains patent because these arterial blood vessels have much thicker walls. This results in venous infarction. Testicular torsion is usually the result of physical trauma in an individual with a predisposing abnormality, such as abnormal development of the gubernaculum testis.

2-15. The answer is c. _(Hardman and Limbird, 9/e, p 1183. Katzung, 7/e, p 785.)_ Fluconazole penetrates into cerebrospinal fluid, where it is active against _Cryptococcus neoformans_. When it is given orally, blood levels are almost as high as when it is given parenterally.

2-16. The answer is a. _(Moore, Embryology 5/e, p 239.)_ Blockage of the foregut in the newborn produces projectile vomiting. Congenital hypertrophic pyloric stenosis, occurring in 0.5 to 1.0 percent of males and rarely in females, involves hypertrophy of the circular layer of muscle at the pylorus. This usually does not regress and must be treated surgically. During the fifth and sixth weeks of development, the lumen of the duodenum is occluded by muscle proliferation, but normally recanalizes during the eighth week. Failure of recanalization results in duodenal atresia. Because this occurs distal to the hepatopancreatic ampulla, the vomitus will occasionally be stained with bile. Annular pancreas, rare in itself, seldom completely blocks the duodenum. Imperforate anus results in intestinal distention with bloating.

2-17. The answer is b. _(Cotran, 5/e, pp 694–699.)_ Acute interstitial pneumonia refers to inflammation of the interstitium of the lung that is the result of infection, typically with either _Mycoplasma pneumoniae_ or viruses, such as influenza A and B. This type of pneumonia is called primary atypical pneumonia because it is "atypical" when compared to the "typical" bacterial pneumonia, such as produced by _Streptococcus pneumoniae_. These bacterial pneumonias are characterized by acute inflammation (neutrophils) within the alveoli. In contrast, acute interstitial pneumonia is characterized by lymphocytes and plasma cells within the interstitium, that is the alveolar septal walls. Viral cytopathic effects, such as inclusion bodies or multinucleated giant cells, may be seen histologically with certain viral infections. Certain viruses produce pneumonia in certain patient groups, that is, respiratory syncytial virus in infants, and adenovirus in military recruits. Infection with _Mycoplasma pneumoniae_ results in the production of a non-specific cold IgM antibody, which characteristically reacts with red cells having the I antigen. Since most adult red cells have I antigens, blood from a patient with mycoplasma pneumonia will hemagglutinate when cooled. This type of reaction is not seen with infection by either *Pneumocystis pneumonia* or *Mycobacteria tuberculosis*.

2-18. The answer is d. *(Fauci, 14/e, p 2427.)* All brain masses are not malignancies. Of these organisms, only *E. coli* has not been described in a cranial mass, and the others are associated with immunodeficiency states.

2-19. The answer is a. *(Nolte, 3/e, pp 356–358.)* The classic appearance of a patient with a lesion of the cerebellar hemispheres is one in which voluntary and skilled movements are affected. They are uncoordinated and there are errors in the range, force, and direction of movement. The relationships between the cerebellum and the motor regions of the cerebral-cortex have been disrupted. Lesions of other regions such as the flocculonodular lobe, vermal region of the anterior cerebellar cortex, or fastigial nucleus produce different symptoms (disturbances of balance, muscle tone, or nystagmus). Although "pure" lesions limited to the ventral spinocerebellar tract have not been reported, it is likely that such a lesion could not account for the symptoms indicated in this question. Information carried by this tract concerns activity of Golgi tendon organs of muscles of the lower limbs.

2-20. The answer is b. *(Cotran, 5/e, pp 1195–1204.)* Psoriasis is a chronic skin disease having large, sharply defined silver-white scaly plaques. These skin lesions are usually found on the extensor surfaces of the elbows and knees, the scalp, and the lumbosacral areas, but additionally about one third of patients have nail changes including discoloration, pitting, and crumbling. The pathogenesis is not well understood, but about one-third of patients have a familial history. The pathogenesis involves a faster turn-over time of the epidermal keratinocytes. The normal turn-over time is about 28 days, but in patients with psoriasis this is decreased to about 3 days. Psoriasis is sometimes associated with other diseases, such as seronegative rheumatoid arthritis and AIDS. Clinically if the scale of psoriasis is lifted, it forms multiple, minute areas of bleeding. This is referred to as an Auspitz sign and is due to increased, dilated vessels within the papillary dermis. The formation of new lesions at sites of trauma is referred to as the Koebner phenomenon, and this sign is also present. In patients with psoriasis, trauma may cause thickening of the epidermis (acanthosis), downward regular elongation of the rete ridges, hyperkeratosis, and parakeratosis. These changes may be related to faulty β-adrenergic receptors and decreased activity of adenyl cyclase in the lower epidermis. Since the keratinocyte turn-over time is faster, there is no granular cell layer. Characteristically, neutrophils infiltrate the epidermis and form Munro's microabscesses in the stratum corneum or Kogoj spongiform pustules in the subcorneal region. These areas within the epidermis are slightly spongiotic, but no bullae are formed. Lymphocytes below a zone of degenerated collagen in the superficial dermis is found in lichen sclerosis, and not psoriasis.

Two bullous diseases that can develop subepidermal bullae are bullous pemphigoid and dermatitis herpetiformis. Bullous pemphigoid is an autoimmune disease that is caused by IgG antibodies to a glycoprotein in the lamina lucida of the basement membrane zone. It is characterized by subepidermal blisters and linear deposits of IgG and C3 in the lamina lucida. Dermatitis herpetiformis is related to gluten sensitivity (celiac disease) and HLA haplotypes B8 and DRw3. Granular deposits of IgA, fibrin, and neutrophils accumulate at the dermal-epidermal junction at the tips of papillae. These changes result in subepidermal vesicles. In patients with systemic lupus erythematosus, patients typically have a malar "butterfly" rash. Histologic examination reveals liquefactive degeneration of the basal layers of the epidermis. Immunoglobulin (IgG) and complement are also deposited at the dermal-epidermal junction in a granular pattern.

2-21. The answer is d. (*Cotran, 5/e, pp 132, 147–148, 449–450. Rubin, 2/e, pp 240–244.*) Several autosomal recessive disorders involve inborn errors of amino acid metabolism. Alkaptonuria (ochronosis) is caused by the excess accumulation of homogentisic acid. This results from a block in the metabolism of the phenylalanine-tyrosine pathway, which is caused by a deficiency of homogentisic oxidase. Excess homogentisic acid causes the urine to turn dark upon standing after a period of time. It also causes a dark coloration of the sclera, tendons, and cartilage. After years, many patients will develop a degenerative arthritis. Phenylketonuria (PKU), also called hyperphenylalaninemia, results from a deficiency of phenylalanine hydroxylase, an enzyme that oxidizes phenylalanine to tyrosine in the liver. Infants are normal at birth, but rising phenylalanine levels (hyperphenylalaninemia) results in irreversible brain damage. The excess phenylacetic acid in the urine results in a "mousy" odor. A lack of the enzyme fumarylacetoacetate hydrolase results in increased levels of tyrosine (tyrosinemia). Chronic forms of the disease are associated with cirrhosis of the liver, kidney dysfunction, and a high risk of developing hepatocellular carcinoma. Maple syrup urine disease is associated with an enzyme defect that causes the accumulation of branched-chain α-keto acid derivatives of isoleucine, leucine, and valine. Albinism refers to a group of disorders characterized by an abnormality of the synthesis of melanin. Two forms of oculocutaneous albinism are classified by the presence or absence of tyrosinase, which is the first enzyme in the conversion of tyrosine to melanin. Albinos are at a greatly increased risk for the development of squamous cell carcinomas in sun-exposed skin.

2-22. The answer is e. *(Hardman and Limbird, 9/e, p 1206. Katzung, 7/e, p 796.)* A major adverse effect of zidovudine is bone marrow depression that appears to be dose- and duration-dependent. The severity of the disease and a low CD4 count contribute to the bone marrow depression.

2-23. The answer is c. *(Adams, 6/e, pp 43–48, 1312–1318.)* This patient does not have an upper motor neuron lesion (spinal cord or above) because of the absent reflexes and ascending paralysis bilaterally involving all of the extremities. Lesions in the brain almost always give unilateral findings, and spinal cord lesions give a distinct level. The damage cannot be in the muscle, because the patient has sensory involvement as well. This case is an example of Guillain-Barré syndrome (GBS), or an inflammatory disease of peripheral nerve resulting from demyelination. Inflammatory cells are found within the nerves, as well as segmental demyelination and some degree of Wallerian degeneration. This damage can cause an ascending paralysis and sensory loss, affecting the arms, face, and legs. The cerebrospinal fluid often has a high protein level, making a spinal tap a useful test for the diagnosis of GBS. Nerve conduction studies are also helpful in making the diagnosis. Most neurologists believe GBS to be an immunologic reaction directed against peripheral nerve, and some patients have a history of some type of infection prior to developing GBS. However, a clear-cut cause is rarely found. Despite a known cause, most patients recover from GBS, although the speed of recovery varies. Treatment is currently available (administration of gamma globulin) and, if instituted early in the course of the disease, decrease in the length of the illness is possible.

2-24. The answer is d. *(Kandel, 3/e, p 386.)* Pain is mediated by C and A-delta fibers in the skin.

2-25. The answer is c. *(Kandel, 3/e, p 368.)* Pacinian corpuscles best mediate vibration.

2-26. The answer is b. *(Adams, 6/e, pp 43–48.)* The reflexes are lost because the lower motor neurons affected by this process are unable to participate in the reflex arc necessary for a knee or ankle jerk to take place. These lower motor neurons originate with stretch receptors in the tendons. Answers A, C, D, and E are all examples of upper motor neuron lesions, usually characterized by hyperactive reflexes.

2-27. The answer is d. *(Fauci, 14/e, p 1982.)* The most definitive and widely accepted test for the diagnosis of acromegaly is the response of growth hormone during an oral glucose tolerance test. Typically, the growth hormone at baseline in acromegaly will be above 5 μg/L. In normal patients, the growth hormone will suppress to less than 2. In acromegalic patients, the growth hormone values may rise, show no change, or suppress partially but not less than 2. A single random growth hormone is not useful, because of the pulsatility in growth hormone. TRH does stimulate growth hormone in many acromegalics but not all. The insulin tolerance test is a stimulation test of growth hormone and not a suppression test.

2-28. The answer is e. *(Gelehrter, pp 159–189. Isselbacher, 13/e, pp 369–371. Jorde, pp 102–105. Thompson, 5/e, pp 201–229.)* Chromosomal abnormalities may involve changes in number (i.e., polyploidy and aneuploidy) or changes in structure (i.e., rearrangements, such as translocations, rings, and inversions). Extra material (i.e., extra chromatin) seen on chromosome 5 implies recombination of chromosome 5 DNA with that of another chromosome to produce a rearranged chromosome. Since this rearranged chromosome 5 takes the place of a normal chromosome 5, there is no change in number of the autosomes (non-sex chromosomes) or sex chromosomes (X and Y chromosomes). The question implies that all cells karyotyped from the patient (usually 11–25 cells) had the same chromosomal constitution, ruling out mosaicism. The patient's clinical findings are similar to those occurring in trisomy 13, suggesting that the extra material on chromosome 5 is derived from chromosome 13, producing an unbalanced karyotype called dup(13) or partial trisomy 13.

2-29. The answer is b. (*Cotran, 5/e, pp 295–297. Chandrasoma, 3/e, pp 858.*) Symptoms not caused by either local or metastatic effects of tumors are called paraneoplastic syndromes. Bronchogenic carcinomas are associated with the development of many different types of paraneoplastic syndromes. These syndromes are usually associated with the secretion of certain substances by the tumor cells. For example, ectopic secretion of ACTH may produce Cushing's syndrome, while ectopic secretion of antidiuretic hormone (syndrome of inappropriate ADH secretion) may produce hyponatremia. Hypocalcemia may result from the production of calcitonin, while hypercalcemia may result from the production of parathyroid hormone-related peptide (PTHrP), which is a normal substance produced locally by many different types of tissue. PTHrP is distinct from parathyroid hormone (PTH). Therefore, patients with this type of paraneoplastic syndrome will have increased calcium levels and decreased PTH levels. As a result of decreased PTH production, all of the parathyroid glands in these patients will be atrophic. Other tumors associated with the production of PTHrP include clear cell carcinomas of the kidney, endometrial adenocarcinomas, and transitional carcinomas of the urinary bladder.

Lung cancers are also associated with multiple, migratory venous thrombosis. This migratory thrombophlebitis is called Trousseau's sign and is more classically associated with carcinoma of the pancreas. Hypertrophic osteoarthropathy is a syndrome consisting of periosteal new bone formation with or without digital clubbing and joint effusion. It is most commonly found in association with lung carcinoma, but it also occurs with other types of pulmonary disease. Erythrocytosis is associated with increased erythropoietin levels and some tumors, particularly renal cell carcinoma, hepatocellular carcinoma, and cerebellar hemangioblastoma. It is not particularly associated with bronchogenic carcinomas.

2-30. The answer is c. (*Alberts, 3/e, p 1216. Coe, pp 803–804. Cotran, 5/e, pp 663–664.*) The patient is suffering from multiple myeloma. In this disease, there are abnormal changes in the bone marrow indicative of altered plasma cell activity and anemia (hemoglobin data and increasing fatigue). These plasma cells produce elevated levels of interleukin 1 (IL-1), which functions as an osteoclast activation factor. The increased IL-1 stimulates osteoclastic activity and results in elevated serum calcium (12.3 mg/dL). The depletion of bone calcium results in lytic lesions of the skull and pelvis as well as the presence of the compression fracture of the spine. The Bence

Jones protein represents free immunoglobulin light chains, which are a diagnostic feature found in the urine of patients with multiple myeloma.

2-31. The answer is a. (*Cotran, 5/e, pp 853, 868–870. Chandrasoma, 3/e, pp 652–653.*) Chronic hepatitis is defined clinically by the presence of elevated serum liver enzymes for longer than 6 months. Liver biopsies in patients with chronic hepatitis may reveal inflammation that is limited to the portal areas (chronic persistent hepatitis), or the inflammation may extend into the adjacent hepatocytes. This inflammation causes necrosis of the hepatocytes (piecemeal necrosis) and is called chronic active hepatitis. These changes are nonspecific and can be seen with hepatitis B virus (HBV) or hepatitis C virus (HCV) infection. The finding of hepatocytes with ground-glass, eosinophilic cytoplasm is highly suggestive of HBV infection, while fatty change (steatosis) is suggestive of HCV. A clinically distinct subtype of chronic hepatitis is called chronic autoimmune ("lupoid") hepatitis. This disease occurs in young females who have no serologic evidence of viral disease. These patients have increased IgG levels and high titers of autoantibodies, such as anti-smooth muscle antibodies and antinuclear antibodies. They also have a positive LE test, which is the basis for the name "lupoid" hepatitis, but there is no relationship of this disease to systemic lupus erythematosus. The prognosis for these patients is poor, as many progress to cirrhosis.

Two diseases classified as primary biliary diseases are primary biliary cirrhosis (PBC) and primary sclerosing cholangitis (PSC). Primary biliary cirrhosis is primarily a disease of middle-aged females and is characterized by pruritus, jaundice, and hypercholesterolemia. More than 90 percent of patients have antimitochondrial autoantibodies, particularly to mitochondrial pyruvate dehydrogenase. A characteristic lesion, called the florid duct lesion, is seen in portal areas and is composed of a marked lymphocytic infiltrate and occasional granulomas. Primary sclerosing cholangitis is characterized by fibrosing cholangitis, which produces concentric "onion-skin fibrosis" in portal areas. It is associated with chronic ulcerative colitis, one type of inflammatory bowel disease.

2-32. The answer is b. (*April, 3/e, pp 579–580.*) The carotid sinus, located at the bifurcation of the common carotid, contains baroceptors. Increased pressure in the carotid body, usually the result of elevated blood pressure but also the result of external pressure, slows and may even arrest the heart.

The carotid body (also at the carotid bifurcation) and the aortic body (lying in the arch of the aorta) contain chemoceptors that monitor the partial pressure of oxygen dissolved in the blood. These are instrumental in initiating the respiratory reflex.

2-33. The answer is e. *(Baum, 3/e, pp 138–148, 275–281.)* Hostility and anger are major triggers for a coronary and increased mortality. The Cook-Medley Hostility Inventory is a scale devised from the hostility components of the Minnesota Multiphasic Personality Inventory (MMPI) and has a high predictability of incidence of coronary heart disease and mortality from all causes.

The Millon Behavioral Health Inventory is a 150-item inventory assessing personality, coping styles, stress, psychosomatic correlates, and indices that predict complications or difficulties with illness. The Cohen Perceived Stress Scale contains a general distress factor, a perceived coping-ability measure, and a scale for symptoms related to depression. The Rosenman and Friedman Type A Structured Interview has a high degree of inter-rater agreement in categorizing people as having Type A or Type B personality characteristics; tense, impatient, hostile, and urgent versus relaxed, quiet, and less hostile, respectively. The Jenkins Activity Survey of Type A behavior is a self-report questionnaire asking about specific Type A behaviors such as hurrying a person along or setting deadlines and quotas that fit the stereotype of the coronary-prone individual. All of the tests listed can provide information on personality factors linked to coronary proneness, but the Cook-Medley Hostility Inventory is the best behavioral predictor because it yields the most accurate data on hostility, the best predicting factor of coronaries and mortality.

2-34. The answer is c. *(Hardman and Limbird, 9/e, p 527. Katzung, 7/e, p 502.)* Naloxone is a pure opioid antagonist at the μ, κ, and δ receptors. μ-Receptor stimulation causes analgesia, euphoria, decreased gastrointestinal (GI) activity, miosis, and respiratory depression. κ-Receptor stimulation causes analgesia, dysphoria, and psychotomimetic effects. δ-Receptor stimulation is not fully understood in humans, but is associated with analgesia and antinociception for thermal stimuli.

2-35. The answer is d. *(Murray, 24/e, pp 242–244. Stryer, pp 624–625.)* Leukotrienes C_4, D_4, and E_4 together compose the slow-reacting substance

(SRS-A) of anaphylaxis, which is thought to be the cause of asphyxiation in individuals not treated rapidly enough following an anaphylactic shock. SRS-A is up to 1000 times more effective in causing bronchial muscle constriction than histamines. Anti-inflammatory steroids are usually given IV to end chronic bronchoconstriction and hypotension following a shock. The steroids block phospholipase A_2 action, preventing the synthesis of leukotrienes from arachidonic acid. Acute treatment involves epinephrine injected subcutaneously initially and then intravenously. Antihistamines such as diphenhydramine are administered intravenously or intramuscularly.

2-36. The answer is d. (*Cotran, 5/e, pp 178–182.*) Hypersensitivity diseases are caused by immune mechanism. They are classified into four different categories based on the immune mechanisms that are involved. Type I hypersensitivity reactions involve IgE (reaginic) antibodies that have been bound to the surface of mast cells and basophils. These IgE antibodies are formed by a T cell dependent process. An allergen initially binds to antigen presenting cells which then activates TH_2 cells to secrete interleukin-4 (IL-4), IL-5, and IL-6. IL-5 stimulates the production of eosinophils, while IL-4 stimulates B cells to transform into plasma cells and produce IgE. This IgE then attaches to mast cells and basophils, because these cells have cell surface receptors for the Fc portion of IgE. When this "armed" mast cell or basophil is re-exposed to the allergen, the antigen bridges two IgE molecules and causes mast cells to release preformed (primary) mediators. This antigen-to-antibody binding also causes these cells to synthesize secondary mediators.

The reactions that occur as a result of the primary mediators of type I hypersensitivity are rapidly occurring since they have already been made and are present within the granules of mast cells. These substances include biogenic amines, such as histamine, chemotactic factors, enzymes, and proteoglycans. Histamine causes increased vascular permeability, vasodilatation, and bronchial smooth muscle contraction. The chemotactic factors are chemotactic for eosinophils and neutrophils. Mast cells will also produce new products (secondary mediators) by a series of reactions within the cell membrane that lead to the generation of lipid mediators and cytokines. The lipid mediators are generated from arachidonic acid. Membrane receptors bound to IgE activate phospholipase A_2, which then cleaves membrane phospholipids into arachidonic acid. Lipoxygenase produces leukotrienes, including LTB4 and the leukotrienes C_4, D_4, and E_4.

These last three leukotrienes are the most potent vasoactive and spasmogenic agents known. They used to be called SRS-A (slow reactive substance of anaphylaxis). Prostaglandin D2, which is produced via the enzyme cyclooxygenase, is abundant in lung mast cells. It causes bronchospasm and increased mucus production.

Type I reactions may be either local reactions or systemic reactions. Local reactions include urticaria ("hives"), angioedema, allergic rhinitis ("hay fever"), conjunctivitis, food allergies, and allergic bronchial asthma. Systemic reactions usually follow parental administration of the antigen, such as with drug reactions (penicillin) or insect stings. The amount of antigen may be very small. Symptoms include vomiting, cramps, diarrhea, itching, wheezing, and shortness of breath, and death may occur within minutes. The main treatment is epinephrine.

2-37. The answer is a. (*Cotran, 5/e, pp 1125–1128.*) Four types of thyroiditis may be associated with hypothyroidism. Hashimoto's thyroiditis, one of the autoimmune thyroid diseases, is associated with the HLA-B8 haplotype and high titers of circulating autoantibodies, including anti-microsomal, anti-thyroglobulin, and anti-TSH receptors antibodies. This abnormality is not that uncommon in the United States.

Histologically there is infiltration of the thyroid stroma by an intense lymphoplasmacytic infiltrate with the formation of lymphoid follicles with germinal centers. This produces destruction and atrophy of the follicles and transforms the thyroid follicular cells into acidophilic cells. There are many different names for these cells, including oxyphilic cells, oncocytes, Hurthle cells, and Askanazy cells. Not uncommonly, patients develop hypothyroidism as a result of follicle disruption, and the manifestations consist of fatigue, myxedema, cold intolerance, hair coarsening, and constipation. Rarely cases of Hashimoto's thyroiditis may develop hyperthyroidism (Hashitoxicosis), while the combination of Hashimoto's disease, pernicious anemia, and type I diabetes mellitus is called Schmidt's syndrome. This is one type of the multiglandular syndromes.

Whereas subacute thyroiditis, Riedel's thyroiditis, and psychosomatic complaints may cause common symptoms, biopsy findings of these disorders are distinctly different from those of Hashimoto's disease. Subacute (DeQuaervain's, granulomatous, or giant cell) thyroiditis is a self-limited viral infection of the thyroid. It typically follows an upper respiratory tract infection. Patients develop the acute onset of fever, painful thyroid enlargement, and may develop a transient hypothyroidism. Histologically there is destruction of the follicles with a granulomatous reaction and multinucleated giant cells that surround fragments of colloid. One-half of the patients with Riedel's thyroiditis are hypothyroid, but in contrast to the other types of thyroiditis, microscopic examination reveals dense fibrosis of the thyroid gland, often extending into extrathyroidal soft tissue. This fibrosis produces a rock-hard enlarged thyroid gland that may produce the feeling of suffocation. This combination of signs and symptoms may be mistaken clinically for a malignant process. Additionally these patients may develop similar fibrosis in the mediastinum or retroperitoneum. Finally, subacute lymphocytic thyroiditis is also a self-limited, painless enlargement of the thyroid that is associated with hypothyroidism, but lacks antithyroid antibodies or lymphoid germinal centers within the thyroid.

2-38. The answer is c. *(Jawetz, 19/e, p 248.)* Pasteurella multocida, a coccobacillary Gram negative rod, is part of the normal mouth flora of dogs and cats. Consequently, many animal bites become infected with this microorganism. It is susceptible to penicillin, although multiresistant strains have been recovered from pigs and sheep. *P. multocida* has four different capsular types—designated A, B, D, and E—that correlate with disease production and host predilection; however, serotyping of these isolates is beyond the resources of most laboratories.

2-39. The answer is d. *(Cotran, 5/e, pp 310, 327–328, 354–357. Rubin, 2/e, pp 408–418.)* Histoplasma capsulatum, a dimorphic fungus, causes one of the three major fungal infections in the United States that may result in systemic infection (Blastomyces and Coccidioides are the other two). Although it commonly produces asymptomatic primary disease, it can result in granulomatous inflammation, especially granulomatous lung disease. Multiple small, yeast surrounded by clear zones may be found within the cytoplasm of macrophages. The source for histoplasma is soil contaminated by the excreta of birds (starlings and chickens) and bats. The typical location for individuals to develop histoplasmosis is the Ohio and Mississippi Valley areas. *Aspergillus* species produce several clinical disease states, including allergic aspergillosis, systemic aspergillosis, and aspergilloma. Typically *Aspergillus* is seen in tissue as acute-angle branching septate hyphae; however, they may form fruiting bodies in cavities, such as within cystic cavities of the lungs. There they may form a large mass called a fungus ball or aspergilloma. Blastomycosis is a chronic granulomatosis disease caused by a dimorphic fungus, *Blastomyces dermatitidis*. In tissues this fungus is seen as a thick walled yeast having broad based budding. Without the budding, *Blastomyces* may be mistaken as cryptococcus. The infection, also known as Gilchrist's disease, is seen in individuals living in the Ohio and Mississippi Valley areas and is usually confined to the lungs. *Candida* species, which frequently cause human infections, grow as yeast, elongated chains of yeast without hyphae (pseudohyphae), or septate hyphae. Mucocutaneous candidal infections can produce white plaques called thrush. Mucormycosis (zygomycosis) is a disease caused by "bread-mold fungi," such as *Rhizopus*, *Mucor*, and *Absidia* species. These infections typically occur in neutropenic patients or diabetics. One form of the disease, typically found in diabetics, is called rhinocerebral mucormycosis and is characterized by facial pain, headache, changing mental status, and a blood-tinged nasal discharge. Tissue sections will reveal characteristic broad, non-septate, right angle branching hyphae.

2-40. The answer is c. (*Kandel, 3/e, p 684. Adams, 6/e, p 89.*) An ataxic gait is an unsteady gait. Gaits due to motor weakness or spasticity tend to involve circling of the weak leg (circumduction), and festinating or shuffling gaits, often due to parkinsonism or disease of the basal ganglia involve a stooped posture with shuffling of the feet and very small steps.

2-41. The answer is d. (*Kandel, 3/e, p 684. Adams, 6/e, pp 89, 118.*) An ataxic gait may result from motor incoordination due to cerebellar disease, or from lack of proprioception in the lower extremities due to disease in the posterior column system (gait becomes unsteady when a patient is unable to detect the location of his/her feet). Degeneration of both systems may occur due to alcoholism, although in this case, we are told that John does not have any sensory deficits when this modality is tested in isolation.

2-42. The answer is b. (*Adams, 6/e, pp 1156–1158.*) This is an example of alcoholic cerebellar degeneration. It is caused by degeneration (probably through nutritional deficiency) of neurons in the cerebellar cortex, particularly of the Purkinje cells, and is usually restricted to anterior and superior parts of the vermis, as well as anterior portions of the anterior lobes. For this reason, most of the deficits in this syndrome involve midline structures such as the trunk, which is represented most in the vermis. Trunk instability usually causes problems with gait. In addition, because the cerebellar homunculus represents the legs in the anterior portion of the anterior lobe, the legs are affected more than the arms. Loss of volume within the vermis of the cerebellum is readily visualized, especially on an MRI of the brain, because this technique allows good visualization of the posterior fossa. If these changes are visualized, then the condition is most likely chronic (as also indicated by the history) and most likely irreversible. However, it is important to make sure that the patient is well nourished, takes vitamins, and stops drinking in order to prevent other neurologic problems from occurring. Damage to other brain regions listed do not cause such damage.

2-43. The answer is b. (*Kandel, 3/e, pp 632–642.*) The spinocerebellum receives sensory inputs from the spinal cord and is instrumental in controlling posture and movement. It includes the vermis and the intermediate hemisphere. The cerebrocerebellum consists of the lateral hemispheres and is instrumental in the planning of movement. The dentate nucleus comprises the cell bodies that form the brachium conjunctivum. The brachium conjunctivum and pontis correspond to the superior and middle cerebellar peduncles, respectively.

2-44. The answer is b. (*Cotran, 5/e, pp 1279, 1336–1338.*) Amyotrophic lateral sclerosis (ALS), Lou Gehrig disease, is a degenerative disorder of motor neurons, principally the anterior horn cells of the spinal cord, the motor nuclei of the brain stem, and the upper motor neurons of the cerebral cortex. Clinically, this disease is a combination of lower motor neuron (LMN) disease with weakness and fasciculations and upper motor neuron (UMN) disease with spasticity and hyperreflexia. Early symptoms include weakness and cramping, then muscle atrophy and fasciculations. Reflexes are hyperactive in upper and lower extremities, and a positive extensor plantar (Babinski) reflex develops because of the loss of upper motor neurons. The triad of atrophic weakness of hands and forearms, slight spasticity of the legs, and generalized hyperreflexia—in the absence of sensory changes—suggests the diagnosis. The clinical course is rapid, and death may result from respiratory complications. There is no effective treatment for ALS. Theories about the etiology of ALS include viral infections, immunologic causes, or oxidative stress. The latter is related to defect in zinc-copper binding superoxide dismutase (SOD) on chromosome 21. Decreased SOD activity leads to apoptosis of spinal motor neurons.

Metachromatic leukodystrophy is an autosomal recessive disorder of sphingomyelin metabolism that results from deficiency of cerebroside sulfatase (aryl-sulfatase A). Sulfatides accumulate in lysosomes and stain metachromatically with cresyl violet. Diagnostic measures include amniocentesis, enzyme analysis, and measuring decreased urinary aryl-sulfatase A. Demyelination is widespread in the cerebrum and peripheral nervous system. Acute inflammatory demyelinating polyradiculoneuropathy (Guillain-Barré syndrome) is a life-threatening disease of the peripheral nervous system. The disease usually follows recovery from an influenza-like upper respiratory tract infection and is characterized by a motor neuropathy that leads to an ascending paralysis which begins with weakness in the distal extremities and rapidly involves proximal muscles. Sensory changes are usually minimal. The disease is thought to result from immune-mediated segmental demyelination. Huntington's disease is characterized by choreiform movements and progressive dementia that appear after the age of 30. Wilson's disease (hepatolenticular degeneration) is an autosomal recessive disorder of copper metabolism in which the total circulating copper is decreased, but the free copper is increased. This leads to athetoid movements, cirrhosis of the liver, and copper deposits in the limbus of the cornea that produce the Kayser-Fleischer ring.

2-45. The answer is c. (*Henry, 19/e, pp 618–620, 626–627, 630–631, 657–659.*) The four main causes of microcytic/hypochromic anemias are iron deficiency, anemia of chronic disease (AOCD), thalassemia, and sideroblastic anemia. Additional laboratory tests can differentiate between these four diseases. The serum iron and percentage of saturation are decreased in both iron deficiency anemia and AOCD, increased in sideroblastic anemia, and may be normal or increased in thalassemia. The total iron-binding capacity (TIBC) is increased only in iron deficiency. It is normal or decreased in the other diseases. An additional differentiating test for these four diagnoses is evaluation of the bone marrow iron stores. In iron deficiency, iron stores are decreased or absent. In AOCD, iron is present, but is restricted to and increased within macrophages. It is decreased in amount within marrow erythroid precursors. Marrow iron is increased in patients with sideroblastic anemia. The iron levels in patients with thalassemia trait are generally within normal limits. Approximately one-third of the normoblasts in the normal bone marrow contain ferritin granules and are called sideroblasts. In sideroblastic anemia, because of the deficiency of pyridoxine and ferritin, the production of globin or heme is markedly reduced, and ferritin granules accumulate within the mitochondria that rim the nucleus. This produces the characteristic ring sideroblast.

2-46. The answer is c. (*Cotran, 5/e, pp 160–161, 506–509, 512.*) Benign tumors of vessels may originate from either blood vessels or lymphatics. Hemangiomas are benign tumors of blood vessels that histologically reveal the presence of red blood cells (erythrocytes) within the lumens of the proliferating vessels. Hemangiomas may be subclassified into capillary hemangiomas or cavernous hemangiomas. The juvenile (strawberry) hemangioma is a fast-growing lesion that appears in the first few months of life, but completely regresses by the age of five. In contrast to hemangiomas, lymphangiomas are tumors that are derived from lymphatic vessels. Histologically they reveal dilated vessels lined by endothelial cells, but they lack red blood cells in their lumen. The absence of red blood cells helps to distinguish these lesions from hemangiomas. Cystic hygromas are cystic lymphangiomas that typically occur in the neck or axilla. They may grow to such a large size that the neck is deformed. These lesions may be found in patients with Turner's syndrome, an abnormality that results from complete or partial monosomy for the X chromosome. Swelling of the neck of these individuals occurs because of dilated lymphatic vessels (cystic hygroma). With time the swelling decreases, but the patients may develop bilateral neck webbing and loose skin on the back of the neck.

Glomangiomas, glomus tumors, are very painful tumors that are derived from the glomus body. These tumors are typically found in the distal regions of the fingers and toes, sometimes in a subungual location. Histologically they reveal vascular spaces that are lined by nests of uniform cells. Dilated blood vessels (vascular ectasia) may be congenital or acquired. "Birthmarks" may be caused by congenital vascular ectasia or capillary hemangiomas. "Port wine stains" are similar lesions that may be caused by vascular ectasia or cavernous hemangiomas of the skin. Spider angiomas are acquired vascular ectasias that are the result of increased estrogen levels. They are associated with pregnancy and liver disease. Bacillary angiomatosis is a non-neoplastic proliferation of blood vessels that is found in immunocompromised patients, particularly patients with AIDS. Histologically there are proliferating capillaries that are lined by protuberant endothelial cells. Additionally numerous neutrophils are present along with nuclear dust and purple granules. These latter granules are rickettsia-like bacteria that are the cause of this lesion, which responds to erythromycin.

2-47. The answer is c. *(McPhee, 2/e, p 6.)* The phenomenon of different phenotypes in individuals with the same genotype is known as variable expressivity. Polymorphism is an allele that is present in 1 percent or more of the population. Mutation refers to an event such as a nucleotide change, deletion, or insertion that produces a new allele. Fitness refers to the ability of an affected individual to reproduce.

2-48. The answer is e. *(Fauci, 14/e, p 1986.)* The suppression of ACTH is characteristic of adrenal adenoma or carcinoma. A CT scan will evaluate for the presence of adrenal tumor. Chest CT is useful in determining ectopic ACTH secretion. An MRI of the pituitary is useful in pituitary-dependent Cushing's disease. The ACTH stimulation test and serum ADH evaluation are not diagnostic in this disease.

2-49. The answer is c. *(Hardman and Limbird, 9/e, p 408.)* Clozapine differs from other neuroleptic agents in that it can induce seizures in nonepileptic patients. In patients with a history of epileptic seizures for which they are not receiving treatment, stimulation of seizures can occur following administration of neuroleptic agents because they lower seizure threshold and cause brain discharge patterns reminiscent of epileptic seizure disorders.

2-50. The answer is e. *(Cotran, 5/e, pp 756–761.)* Most lesions of the esophagus present with similar symptoms, such as heartburn and dysphagia, but the most serious disease, which carries the risk of exsanguination, is bleeding esophageal varices. Varices occur in about two-thirds of all patients with cirrhosis, and in the majority of patients the etiology is alcoholic cirrhosis. The cirrhosis causes portal hypertension, which shunts blood into connecting channels between the portal and caval systems, such as the subepithelial plexus of veins in the lower esophagus. Varices produce no symptoms until they rupture and cause massive bleeding (hematemesis), which may lead to death. Other diseases may cause hematemesis such as gastritis, esophageal laceration (Mallory-Weiss tears), or peptic ulcer disease. Dysphagia (difficulty swallowing) is another esophageal symptom.

It is seen in diseases with abnormal esophageal function, such as achalasia, and diseases that narrow the esophageal lumen, such as webs and rings. The characteristics of achalasia include aperistalsis, incomplete relaxation of the lower esophageal sphincter (LES) with swallowing, and increased resting tone of the LES, all of which lead to esophageal dilatation and symptoms of progressive dysphagia. Plummer-Vinson syndrome is the combination of esophageal webs in the upper esophagus and anemia. Outpouchings in the upper esophagus are called pharyngeal (Zenker's) diverticuli and may result in regurgitation and aspiration. Sliding hiatal hernias are associated with signs and symptoms of reflux esophagitis.

BLOCK 3

Answers

3-1. The answer is c. *(April, 3/e, p 57.)* The clavicle is very susceptible to fracture because its S-shape produces strong shear forces in the central third during a fall on an outstretched arm. The facts that the clavicle is the first bone in the body to begin the ossification process and usually the last to complete that process are not related to the high incidence of clavicular fracture. Likewise, neither the subcutaneous location nor the strong acromioclavicular and sternoclavicular joints contribute significantly to the high incidence of fracture.

3-2. The answer is d. *(Damjanov, 10/e, pp 1125–1144. Rubin, 2/e, p 1033.)* Clinicians and pathologists alike should be familiar with the benign syndrome of lymph node enlargement called sinus histiocytosis with massive lymphadenopathy. This is a self-limiting, invariably benign disorder found classically in young, black, African and Caribbean patients, but it has been found in others as well. It is characterized clinically by profound enlargement of regional cervical lymph nodes, fever, and leukocytosis. Histologically, the lymph nodes show marked histiocytic proliferation within the sinuses, with engulfment of lymphocytes within the histiocytes. There may be skin involvement, and histiocytes containing phagocytosed lymphocytes may be present in the skin biopsy specimen. The patients predictably revert to normal within a period of months. Histiocytic medullary reticulosis is a disease in which a form of malignant histiocytes is found in lymph node sinuses, with engulfed red cells found within the neoplastic histiocytes (erythrophagocytosis). Primitive, round lymphoblastic tumor cells are found in tissue taken from patients with Burkitt's lymphoma.

3-3. The answer is e. *(Cotran, 5/e, pp 520–523.)* The morphological changes of clinical congestive heart failure cannot always be correlated with necropsy findings of the heart because there may be hypertrophy, dilatation, a combination of both, or even an absence of both. Many patients with long-standing congestive heart failure after decompensation will have hearts that are maximally dilated, with thinned and unusually soft myocardium rather than hypertrophic ventricular myocardium. This thinning of the myocardium occurs after a long period of compensatory hypertrophy and reflects a state in which the capacity of the myocardium to compensate has been exceeded. The first response of the myocardium to a demand for increased work (load) is to undergo hypertrophy according to Starling's law, leading to an increase in stroke volume. Eventually, this mechanism is exceeded under states of increased oxygen demand or demand for more cardiac output, and cardiac decompensation results, with the worst complication being acute pulmonary edema as a consequence of left ventricular failure.

3-4. The answer is c. *(Cotran, 5/e, pp 1144–1147. Rubin, 2/e, pp 1126–1128.)* Parathyroid hyperplasia may be associated with either primary or secondary hyperparathyroidism. In contrast to primary hyperparathyroidism, secondary hyperparathyroidism results from hypocalcemia and causes secondary hypersecretion of parathyroid hormone (PTH). This results in the combination of hypocalcemia and increased PTH. This abnormality is principally found in patients with chronic renal failure where phosphate retention is thought to cause hypocalcemia. Since the failing kidney is not able to synthesize 1,25-dihydroxycholecalciferol, the most active form of vitamin D, this deficiency leads to poor absorption of calcium from the gut and relative hypocalcemia, which stimulates excess PTH secretion. Chronic renal failure is the most important cause, but secondary hyperparathyroidism also occurs in vitamin D deficiency, malabsorption syndromes, and pseudohypoparathyroidism. In any of the causes of parathyroid hyperplasia all four parathyroid glands are typically enlarged. Parathyroid hyperplasia can be differentiated from parathyroid adenomas by the fact that parathyroid hyperplasia, either primary or secondary, results in enlargement of all four glands, while a parathyroid adenoma or parathyroid carcinoma will produce enlargement of only one gland. In most cases the other three glands are smaller than normal.

3-5. The answer is a. *(Fauci, 14/e, p 1976.)* Established therapy of hyperprolactinemia from a pituitary adenoma is treatment with a dopamine agonist, such as bromocriptine. Surgical therapy usually does not result in a cure in a macroadenoma and is reserved for those patients who are intolerant to dopamine agonist. Transfrontal surgery is rarely utilized. Somatostatin agonist and thyroxine have little effect on hyperprolactinemia.

3-6. The answer is b. (*Davis, 4/e, pp 548–549.*) Toxic shock syndrome (TSS) is a febrile illness seen predominantly, but not exclusively, in menstruating women. Clinical criteria for TSS include fever greater than 102°F (38.9°C), rash, hypotension, and abnormalities of the mucous membranes and the gastrointestinal, hepatic, muscular, cardiovascular, or central nervous system. Usually three or more systems are involved. Treatment is supportive, including the aggressive use of antistaphylococcal antibiotics. Certain types of tampons may play a role in TSS by trapping O_2 and depleting magnesium. Most people have protective antibodies to the toxic shock syndrome toxin (TSST-1).

Toxic shock syndrome (TSS) is caused by a toxin-producing strain of *Staphylococcus aureus* (TSST-1). While there have been reports that *S. epidermidis* produces TSS, they have largely been discounted. Vaginal colonization with *S. aureus* is a necessary adjunct to the disease. *S. aureus* is isolated from the vaginal secretions, conjunctiva, nose, throat, cervix, and feces in 45 to 98 percent of cases. The organism has infrequently been isolated from the blood.

3-7. The answer is d. (*Adams, 6/e, pp 321–322.*) This is an example of a complex partial seizure, most likely originating in the temporal lobe. A seizure is a paroxysmal derangement of the central nervous system due to rhythmic, synchronous discharges from cerebral neurons, causing changes in consciousness, sensation and/or behavior. Complex partial seizures often start with a warning or "aura." Since limbic structures are often involved, the seizure can include emotions, feelings of deja-vu or jamais-vu, or gastrointestinal sensations. Because olfactory pathways end in the temporal lobe, patients may experience "smells" as well. The seizure itself involves impairment of consciousness of some form, often manifested as staring, in addition to various stereotyped, automatic behaviors called *automatisms*. The latter may be manifested as chewing, repetitive swallowing, hand gestures, or vocalizations. These usually occur during the seizure, but may occur after it. After the seizure ends (the seizures usually last 1 to 2 minutes), the patient is often in a confused or postictal state for several minutes, or even up to several hours. Occasionally, a patient may manifest aggressive behavior while in the postictal state. Unless a structural lesion, such as a tumor, is present, the physical examination is usually normal. Verification of the diagnosis of epilepsy is done with the help of an electroencephalogram, or EEG, which records potential differences of summed cortical action potentials over the scalp of a patient. Often, an epileptic spike, or sharp wave, is seen over the area from which the seizures arise. Epilepsy patients usually also have a CT scan or MRI (magnetic resonance imaging) to make certain that there is no structural lesion causing the seizures.

3-8. The answer is c. *(Adams, 6/e, pp 321–322.)* Seizures similar to this one often begin with abnormal neuronal discharges in temporal lobe structures, which include the amygdala or hippocampus. These structures tend to have a lower threshold for this type of activity than other structures in the brain.

3-9. The answer is d. *(Kandel, 3/e, p 737.)* The major descending pathways from the amygdala are the stria terminalis and the ventral amygdalofugal pathway. The medial forebrain bundle is a major pathway of the lateral hypothalamus. The mamillothalamic and corticospinal tracts do not involve the amygdala.

3-10. The answer is a. *(Kandel, 3/e, p 737.)* The hippocampal formation includes the hippocampus, the dentate gyrus, and the subiculum. All of the other structures listed are within the limbic system, but do not lie within the hippocampal formation.

3-11. The answer is c. *(Cotran, 5/e, pp 31–32, 858.)* Hyaline is a non-specific term that is used to describe any material, inside or outside the cell, that stains a red homogenous color with the routine hematoxylin and eosin (H&E) stain. There are many different substances that have the appearance of hyaline. Alcoholic hyaline inclusions (Mallory bodies) are irregular eosinophilic hyaline inclusions that are found within the cytoplasm of hepatocytes. Mallory bodies are composed of prekeratin intermediate filaments. They are a nonspecific finding and can be found in patients with several diseases other than alcoholic hepatitis, such as Wilson's disease, and bypass operations for morbid obesity. Immunoglobulins may form intracytoplasmic or extracellular oval hyaline bodies called Russell bodies. Excess plasma proteins may form hyaline droplets in proximal renal tubular epithelial cells or hyaline membranes in the alveoli of the lungs (hyaline membrane disease). The hyaline found in the walls of arterioles of kidneys in patients with benign nephrosclerosis is composed of basement membranes and precipitated plasma proteins. Lipofuscin is an intracytoplasmic aging pigment that has a yellow-brown, finely granular appearance with H&E stains. Its appearance does not resemble hyaline material.

3-12. The answer is b. *(Hardman and Limbird, 9/e, p 1299. Katzung, 7/e, p 925.)* Nephrotoxicity may occur in almost three-quarters of patients treated with cyclosporine. Regular monitoring of blood levels can reduce the incidence of adverse effects.

3-13. The answer is d. *(McPhee, 2/e, p 5.)* Given a set of defined criteria, recognition of the condition in individuals known to carry the mutated gene is described as penetrance. Reduced penetrance is commonly seen in dominantly inherited conditions that have relatively high fitness, such as Huntington's disease or polycystic kidney disease.

3-14. The answer is a. *(Cotran, 5/e, pp 557–562.)* Cardiomyopathies can be separated into a dilated form, a hypertrophic form, a restrictive form, and an obliterative form. In hypertrophic cardiomyopathy, also called idiopathic hypertrophic subaortic stenosis (IHSS), and asymmetric septal hypertrophy (ASH), the major gross abnormality is within the interventricular septum. There is asymmetric hypertrophy of the septum, which is thicker than the left ventricle. Histologically, the myofibers in the septum are disorganized, hypertrophied, and have hyperchromatic nuclei. There is an increased incidence of hypertrophic cardiomyopathy within families, and there is evidence that it may be an autosomal dominant disorder. The disease is thought to result from a mutation in the cardiac β-myosin heavy chain gene. Patients may have dyspnea, light-headedness, and chest pain, especially upon physical exertion; however, many patients appear to be asymptomatic. Up to one-third of these patients die from sudden cardiac death, usually related to physical exertion. Cardiac output can be markedly reduced in some patients because of reduced volume of the left ventricle.

Patients with dilated (congestive) cardiomyopathy have a flabby, hypocontractile heart. Constrictive (restrictive) cardiomyopathy is associated in the United States with amyloidosis and endocardial fibroelastosis. It is so named because of the infiltration and deposition of material in the endomyocardium and the layering of collagen and elastin over the endocardium. This deposition affects the ability of the ventricles to accommodate blood volume during diastole. Endocardial fibroelastosis occurs mainly in infants during the first two years of life. It is associated with a prominent fibroelastic covering over the endocardium of the left ventricle. There may be associated aortic coarctation, ventricular septal defects, mitral valve defects, and other abnormalities. In contrast, endomyocardial fibrosis is a form of restrictive cardiomyopathy that is found mainly in young adults and children in Southeast Asia and Africa. It differs from endocardial fibroelastosis in the United States in that elastic fibers are not present.

3-15. The answer is a. *(Cotran, 5/e, pp 1144–1147. Chandrasoma, 3/e, pp 857–863.)* Hyperparathyroidism is caused by excess production of parathyroid hormone (PTH). In patients with hyperparathyroidism it is important to distinguish primary hyperparathyroidism from secondary hyperparathyroidism. Both forms may be associated with the development of bone lesions, but excess PTH production in primary hyperparathyroidism leads to different laboratory values than those seen with secondary hyperparathyroidism. Increased levels of PTH in primary hyperparathyroidism result in the following laboratory results: increased serum calcium (hypercalcemia) and decreased serum phosphorus. The serum calcium levels are elevated because of increased bone resorption and increased intestinal calcium absorption, the result of increased activity of vitamin D. PTH also increases calcium reabsorption in the distal renal tubule, but because the filtered load of calcium exceeds the ability for reabsorption, calcium is increased in the urine (hypercalciuria). PTH also increases the urinary excretion of phosphate. The excess calcium in the urine predisposes to renal stone formation, especially calcium oxalate or calcium phosphate stones. Urinary stones can produce flank pain and hematuria. This is the most common presentation for patients with hyperparathyroidism. The hypercalcemia of hyperparathyroidism may also cause peptic ulcer disease, which is due to the stimulation of gastrin release and increased acid secretion from the parietal cells. The hypercalcemia also results in muscle weakness, fatigue, and hypomotility of the GI tract, which can lead to constipation and nausea. Alterations of mental status are also common.

In contrast to primary hyperparathyroidism, secondary hyperparathyroidism results from hypocalcemia. This causes secondary hypersecretion of PTH and produces the combination of hypocalcemia and increased PTH production. It is primarily found in patients with chronic renal failure. Patients with hypoparathyroidism develop hypocalcemia, hyperphosphatemia, but have normal serum creatinine levels. Primary hypoparathyroidism and pseudohypoparathyroidism also result in decreased 24-hour excretion of calcium and phosphate.

3-16. The answer is a. *(Cotran, 5/e, p 1334.)* Huntington's disease, an autosomal dominant disorder that results from an abnormal gene on chromosome 4, involves the extrapyramidal system and atrophy of the caudate nuclei and putamen. Choreiform movements and progressive dementia appear after the age of 30. There is degeneration of GABA neurons in the striatum, which leads to decreased function (decreased inhibition) and increased movement. Huntington's disease is one of four diseases that are characterized by long repeating sequences of three nucleotides (the other diseases being fragile X syndrome, myotonic dystrophy, and spinal and bulbar muscular atrophy). Therapy for excessive movement (hyperkinetic) disorders can be attempted with dopamine antagonists. Decreased dopamine in the striatum theoretically will cause a relative increase in acetylcholine and an increase in excitation in the striatum. This will cause increased GABA function, which leads to increased inhibition of movement. The same result could theoretically be achieved with inhibition of acetylcholine breakdown (cholinesterase inhibitors). Compare this to the same treatment of hypokinetic (Parkinson) disorders. Dopamine agonists will increase the inhibition in the striatum, which will lead to decreased GABA in the striatum and decreased inhibition of movement (increased movement). The same result could theoretically be achieved with anticholinergics.

3-17. The answer is d. (*McPhee, 2/e, pp 481 and 532–534; Fauci 14/e, pp 2021–2023.*) Hypothyroidism is the cause of this patient's amenorrhea. Classic findings of hypothyroidism presented here are increased cold intolerance, loss of energy, and hair and weight gain. The best test for this disorder is that for TSH.

3-18. The answer is a. (*Damjanov, 10/e, pp 714–716. Cotran, 5/e, pp 327–328.*) Protein-calorie malnutrition in underdeveloped countries leads to a spectrum of symptoms from kwashiorkor at one end to marasmus at the other. Marasmus, caused by a lack of caloric intake (i.e., starvation), leads to generalized wasting, stunted growth, atrophy of muscles, and loss of subcutaneous fat. There is no edema or hepatic enlargement. These children are alert, not apathetic, and are ravenous. In contrast, children with kwashiorkor, which is characterized by a lack of protein despite adequate caloric intake, have peripheral edema, a "moon" face, and an enlarged, fatty liver. The peripheral edema is caused by decreased albumin and sodium retention, while the fatty liver is caused by decreased synthesis of the lipoproteins necessary for the normal mobilization of lipids from liver cells. Additionally these children have "flaky paint" areas of skin and abnormal pigmented streaks in their hair ("flag sign"). In children with marasmus, the skin is inelastic due to loss of subcutaneous fat. In either severe kwashiorkor or marasmus, thymic atrophy may result in the reduction in number and function of circulating T cells. B-cell function (i.e., immunoglobulin production) is also depressed, so that these children are highly vulnerable to infections.

3-19. The answer is b. (*Cotran, 5/e, pp 1071–1077. Chandrasoma, 3/e, pp 775–776.*) Ovarian neoplasms are divided into four main categories: epithelial tumors, sex cord-stromal tumors, germ cell tumors, and metastases. Examples of ovarian stromal tumors include thecomas, fibromas, granulosa cell tumors, and Sertoli-Leydig cell tumors. Histologically thecomas are composed of spindle-shaped cells with vacuolated cytoplasm. They are vacuolate because of steroid hormone (estrogen) production, which can be stained with an oil red O stain. Fibromas are also composed of spindle-shaped cells, but they do not produce steroid hormones and are oil red O negative. Fibromas are associated with Meig's syndrome, which consists of an ovarian fibroma, ascites, and hydrothorax. Granulosa cell tumors vary in the clinical behavior, but they are considered to be potentially malignant. The stromal cells of the ovary are the precursors of endocrine active cells, so it is easy to understand that neoplasms derived from these stromal cells are often associated with hormone production. For example, granulosa cells normally secrete estrogens, thecal cells normally secrete androgens, and hilar cells (Leydig cells) may secrete androgens. Excess androgen production in females may lead to masculinization and produce symptoms such as amenorrhea, loss of secondary female sex characteristics, and the development of secondary male characteristics, such as hirsutism, temporal balding, and deepening of the voice. Ovarian tumors associated with excess androgen production include androblastomas (Sertoli-Leydig cell tumors). Other ovarian diseases associated with excess androgen production include polycystic ovarian disease and hyperthecosis. Excess estrogen production is associated with precocious puberty in the young, or endometrial hyperplasia and cancer in older women. Ovarian tumors that may secrete estrogens include granulosa cell tumors and thecomas.

3-20. The answer is d. (*Hardman and Limbird, 9/e, pp 404–406.*) Although most antipsychotic agents can cause orthostatic hypotension, thioridazine is the most likely choice of the agents above for causing this adverse effect.

3-21. The answer is d. *(Gelehrter, pp 39–44. Isselbacher, 13/e, pp 346–347. Jorde, pp 86–96. Scriver, 7/e, pp 76–78. Thompson, 5/e, pp 72–82.)* When evaluating the possibility of an X-linked disorder, it is important to remember the pattern of inheritance of the X chromosome. Females have two X chromosomes, which are passed along in a random fashion. They will pass any given X chromosome to 50 percent of their sons and 50 percent of their daughters. For a recessive condition, those daughters who inherit the affected allele will be heterozygous carriers of the disorder but will not be affected. Since males have only one X chromosome, those who inherit the affected allele will be affected with the disorder.

3-22. The answer is d. *(Fauci, 14/e, p 346.)* *Pseudomonas* is not associated with nonmalignant lymphadenopathy.

3-23. The answer is b. *(Cotran, 5/e, pp 867–871. Rubin, 2/e, pp 740–744.)* Diseases of the biliary tract may lead to manifestations of jaundice and if prolonged and severe may lead to cirrhosis. These diseases can be classified as either primary or secondary. Causes of secondary biliary cirrhosis include biliary atresia, gallstones, and carcinoma of the head of the pancreas. Histologic examination of the liver may reveal bile stasis in the interlobular bile ducts and bile duct proliferation in the portal areas. Primary biliary cirrhosis (PBC) is primarily a disease of middle-aged women and is characterized by pruritus, jaundice, and hypercholesterolemia. More than 90 percent of patients have antimitochondrial autoantibodies, particularly the "M2" antibody to mitochondrial pyruvate dehydrogenase. A characteristic lesion, called the florid duct lesion, is seen in portal areas and is composed of a marked lymphocytic infiltrate and occasional granulomas. Primary sclerosing cholangitis (PSC) is characterized by fibrosing cholangitis that produces concentric "onion-skin" fibrosis in portal areas. It is highly associated with chronic ulcerative colitis. Abnormal development of the biliary tract may lead to several abnormalities, including von Meyenburg's complex (small bile duct hamartomas near normal portal tracts) and Caroli's disease, which is characterized by segmental dilatation of the larger intrahepatic bile ducts.

3-24. The answer is b. *(Stryer, 4/e, p 472.)* In many populations, a majority of adults are deficient in lactase and hence intolerant to the lactose in milk. In all populations, at least some adults have this deficiency. Since virtually all children are able to digest lactose, this deficiency develops in adulthood. In such lactase-deficient adults, lactose accumulates in the small intestine because no transports exist for the disaccharide. An outflow of water into the gut owing to the osmotic effect of the milk sugar causes the clinical symptoms. Steatorrhea, or fatty stools, is caused by unabsorbed fat, which can occur following a fatty meal in persons with a deficiency of lipoprotein lipase.

3-25. The answer is d. (*Cotran, 5/e, pp 242–244. Chandrasoma, 3/e, pp 264–268.*) The names given to tumors are based on the parenchymal component of the tumor, which consists of the proliferating neoplastic cells. In general benign tumors are designated by using the suffix "-oma" attached to a name describing either the cell of origin of the tumor or the gross or microscopic appearance of the tumor. Examples of naming benign tumors based on their microscopic appearance include adenomas, which have a uniform proliferation of glandular epithelial cells, papillomas, which are tumors that form finger-like projections, fibromas, which are composed of a uniform proliferation of fibrous tissue, hemangiomas, which are formed from a uniform proliferation of endothelial cells, and lipomas, which originate from adipocytes. The suffix "-oma" is unfortunately still applied to some tumors that are not benign. Examples of this misnaming include melanomas, lymphomas, and seminomas.

Malignant tumors are generally classified as being either carcinomas or sarcomas. Carcinomas are malignant tumors of epithelial origin, while sarcomas are malignant tumors of mesenchymal tissue. Examples of malignant epithelial tumors (carcinomas) include adenocarcinomas, which consist of a disorganized mass of malignant cells that form glandular structures, and squamous cell carcinomas, which consist of a disorganized mass of malignant cells that produce keratin. Examples of malignant mesenchymal tumors include leiomyosarcomas, fibrosarcomas, and liposarcomas. One clue that a tumor developed from skeletal muscle is the presence of cross-striations. These individual cells seen histologically are called "strap cells." The wall of the stomach consists of smooth muscle, and a tumor that originates from these smooth muscle cells will consist of proliferating cells with elongated, spindle-shaped nuclei. If this tumor is benign it will be called a leiomyoma, while if it is malignant it will be called a leiomyosarcoma. This distinction is based on the number of mitoses that are present and the degree of atypia displayed by the neoplastic cells.

3-26. The answer is c. (*Damjanov, 10/e, pp 1089, 1716, 1751, 1823. Cotran, 5/e, pp 619–620, 980–981.*) A woman who manifests a hemorrhagic diathesis following childbirth should be considered to have intravascular coagulopathy until proof to the contrary is obtained—for instance, the condition may be due to retained products of conception. However, the peripheral blood smear depicted in the question shows, in addition to thrombocytopenia (three to four platelets are normally present in every high-power field), remarkably misshapen red blood cells (poikilocytosis) in the form of schistocytes (fragments of red cells), spherocytes, and, importantly, "helmet" red cells, so named because of their similarity in shape to military or football helmets. Helmet cells imply the presence of microangiopathic hemolytic anemia and are thought to form through hemolytic-mechanical red cell membrane disruption by passing through arteriole-capillary beds that have fibrin thrombin meshes. Disorders that cause microangiopathic hemolytic anemia are childhood and adult hemolytic uremic syndrome and thrombotic thrombocytopenic purpura (TTP). The lack of jaundice and neurologic symptoms in this case rules out TTP. The combination of microangiopathic hemolytic anemia and renal insufficiency strongly suggests hemolytic uremic syndrome.

3-27. The answer is a. (*Jawetz, 19/e, pp 452–467.*) The *e* antigen seems to be related to the Dane particle, which is presumed to be the intact hepatitis B virus. Possession of the *e* antigen suggests active disease and, thus, an increased risk of transmission of hepatitis to others. HBsAg and *e* antigen are components of hepatitis B and are not shared by other hepatitis viruses.

3-28. The answer is a. (*McPhee, 2/e, pp 557–558; Fauci, 14/e, pp 262–265.*) Detrusor instability, decreased contractility, and failure are all part of a continuum. Decreased contractility is implied by the decreased force of the stream. Instability alone has only frequency and urgency. Failure implies an inability to urinate due to muscle failure. With acute obstruction, the patient cannot void, and there is significant pain. With chronic urinary obstruction, starting the stream is also a problem.

3-29. The answer is a. (*Cotran, 5/e, p 156. Rubin, 2/e, p 220.*) Several genetic diseases are characterized by a deletion of part of an autosomal chromosome. The 5p⁻ syndrome is also called the cri du chat syndrome as affected infants characteristically have a high-pitched cry similar to that of a kitten. Additional findings in this disorder include severe mental retardation, microcephaly, and congenital heart disease. The 11p⁻ syndrome is characterized by the congenital absence of the iris (aniridia) and is often accompanied by Wilms tumor of the kidney. The 13q⁻ syndrome is associated with the loss of the Rb suppressor gene and the development of retinoblastoma. Signs and symptoms of patients with either 21q⁻ or 22q⁻ are similar to those of Down's syndrome.

3-30. The answer is c. (*Hardman and Limbird, 9/e, p 340. Katzung, 7/e, p 426.*) Of the listed agents, only bupivacaine is an amide. Allergy to amide-type local anesthetics is much less frequent than with ester-type local anesthetics, such as benzocaine; patients who demonstrate allergy to one such drug will be allergic to all of them.

3-31. The answer is a. (*Junqueira, 8/e, pp 315–316, 320–322. Ross, 3/e, pp 497, 506–507.*) Bilirubin, a product of iron-free heme, is liberated during the destruction of old erythrocytes by the mononuclear macrophages of the spleen and, to a lesser extent, of the liver and bone marrow. The hepatic portal system brings splenic bilirubin to the liver, where it is made soluble for excretion by conjugation with glucuronic acid. Commonly, initial low levels of glucuronyl transferase in the underdeveloped smooth endoplasmic reticulum of hepatocytes in the newborn result in jaundice (neonatal hyperbilirubinemia); less commonly, this enzyme is genetically lacking. The ability of mature hepatocytes to take up and conjugate bilirubin may be exceeded by abnormal increases in erythrocyte destruction (hemolytic jaundice) or by hepatocellular damage (functional jaundice), such as in hepatitis. Finally, obstruction of the duct system between the liver and duodenum (usually of the common bile duct in the adult and rarely from aplasia of the duct system in infants) results in a backup of bilirubin (obstructive jaundice). However, obstruction of the cystic duct, while painful, will not interfere with the flow of bile from the liver to the duodenum.

3-32. The answer is b. (*Cotran, 5/e, pp 703–706, 714–715.*) Interstitial pulmonary fibrosis (IF) may be a slowly progressive disease with no recognizable etiology. This disease entity has many names, such as chronic interstitial pneumonitis and diffuse fibrosing alveolitis, but the common name is usual interstitial pneumonitis (UIP). The form of this disease that progresses very rapidly is called the Hamman-Rich syndrome. The pathogenesis of UIP involves damage to type I pneumocytes with the subsequent proliferation of type II pneumocytes and secretion of factors by macrophages that cause fibrosis. The end stage form of IF is characterized by large cysts with intervening fibrosis, which imparts the gross appearance of a "honeycomb lung." There are several subtypes of IF which are characterized by their histologic appearance. Lymphocytic interstitial pneumonitis (LIP) has numerous lymphocytes, Giant cell interstitial pneumonitis (GIP) has giant cells, and plasma cell interstitial pneumonitis (PIP) has numerous plasma cells. LIP is seen in patients with Sjögren's syndrome or AIDS and is associated with an increased risk of developing lymphoma. An important subtype is desquamative interstitial pneumonitis (DIP), which is characterized histologically by sheets of cells within the alveoli. This type of IF may respond to the use of steroids. UIP, in contrast, does not respond to therapy, and therefore treatment is symptomatic treatment only. Theophylline is used to treat asthma, antibiotics are used to treat bacterial infections, and INH is used in combination with other drugs to treat tuberculosis.

3-33. The answer is b. (*Cotran, 5/e, pp 98, 616–617. Isselbacher, 13/e, pp 305–306.*) Hemorrhages into the skin may produce lesions of varying sizes. Petechiae measure less than 2 mm in size, purpuric lesions measure 2 mm to 1 cm, and ecchymoses are larger than 1 cm. Both erythema and telangiectasis do not involve hemorrhage outside of blood vessels. They can be differentiated from true hemorrhages into the skin by the fact that they will blanch if direct pressure is applied to them. True purpura may be caused by hemostatic defects or non-hemostatic defects. Hemostatic defects are caused by platelet or coagulation abnormalities, while non-hemostatic defects generally involve the blood vessels. These vascular abnormalities can be separated into palpable and nonpalpable purpura. The latter may be caused by excess corticosteroids (Cushing's syndrome), vitamin C deficiency (scurvy), infectious agents, and abnormal connective tissue diseases (Ehlers-Danlos syndrome). Causes of palpable purpura include diseases that cause cutaneous vasculitis, such as collagen vascular diseases and Henoch-Schönlein purpura. The latter, also known as anaphylactoid purpura, is a type of hypersensitivity vasculitis found in children. It usually develops one to three weeks following a streptococcal infection, but it may also occur in relation to allergic food reactions. Cross-reacting IgA or immune complexes are deposited on the endothelium of blood vessels.

Patients may develop fever, purpura, abdominal pain, arthralgia, arthritis, and glomerulonephritis.

3-34. The answer is d. *(Davis, 4/e, pp 869, 893–894.)* Recurrent severe infection is an indication for clinical evaluation of immune status. Live vaccines, including BCG attenuated from *Mycobacterium tuberculosis*, should not be used in the evaluation of a patient's immune competence because patients with severe immunodeficiencies may develop an overwhelming infection from the vaccine. For the same reason, oral (Sabin) polio vaccine is not advisable for use in such persons.

3-35. The answer is b. *(Katzung, 7/e, p 773.)* Rifampin induces P-450 enzymes, which causes a significant increase in elimination of drugs such as oral contraceptives, anticoagulants, ketoconazole, cyclosporine, and chloramphenicol. It also promotes urinary excretion of methadone, which may precipitate withdrawal.

3-36. The answer is c. *(Cotran, 5/e, pp 310, 355. Rubin, 2/e, pp 408–418.)* Cryptococcosis is caused by *Cryptococcus neoformans*, an encapsulated yeast (not dimorphic) that infects the central nervous system, primarily in immunocompromised patients. The soil-dwelling yeast is inhaled, but lung involvement tends to be mild in individuals that are not immunodeficient. Diagnosis of cryptococcal meningitis is achieved by finding encapsulated yeasts in CSF preparations. The capsule can be seen with a mucicarmine stain, or it can be negatively stained using India ink. The CSF and serum should also be tested for cryptococcal antigen by the latex cryptococcal agglutination test (LCAT), which is positive in more than 90 percent of cases. Cryptococcal meningitis varies from a chronic inflammatory and granulomatous infection to a noninflammatory meningitis with numerous yeasts massed, sometimes forming cystic "soap bubble" lesions in the brain. Do not confuse cryptococcus with cryptosporidium. *Cryptosporidium parvum* is a protozoan parasite that may cause a transient diarrhea in immunocompetent individuals or a chronic diarrhea in patients with AIDS (cryptosporidiosis). Histologically, sporozoites may be found attached to the surface of intestinal epithelial cells. They are best seen with an acid-fast stain. Chromomycosis is a chronic infection of the skin that is produced by an organism that appears as a brown thick-walled sphere ("copper penny") in tissue sections. Coccidiomycosis is a mycotic infection caused by inhalation of the arthrospores of the dimorphic fungus *Coccidioides immitis*. Within the lung the spores enlarge to from large spherules (sporangia) that become filled with many small endospores. The cyst will rupture, releasing the endospores. Unruptured spherules incite a granulomatous reaction, while the endospores cause a neutrophilic response. Paracoccidiomycosis (South American blastomycosis) is a chronic granulomatous infection caused by *Paracoccidioides brasiliensis*, a dimorphic fungus seen in tissues as a large central organism having peripheral oval budding. This histologic appearance is described as being similar to a mariner's wheel.

3-37. The answer is d. (*Cotran, 5/e, pp 329–334, 790–794, 804–806.*) Early stages of ulcerative colitis (UC) may be indistinguishable from gastroenteritis caused by *Salmonella choleraesuis* and *S. typhimurium*. In early stages, both diseases may show histologically a dense mononuclear inflammatory infiltrate in the lamina propria, occasional crypt abscesses, and mucosal edema and congestion. Even the respective clinical symptoms and colon x-ray changes may be similar, although marked vomiting should point to food poisoning. Salmonellae have been the cause of outbreaks and epidemics of acute gastroenteritis, and the cause has often been found to be contaminated fowl that has been insufficiently cooked to inactivate endotoxins.

3-38. The answer is e. (*Noback, 5/e, p 261. Nolte, 3/e, pp 356–358.*) Since the flocculonodular lobe receives and integrates inputs from the vestibular system, it is understandable why lesions that disrupt this integrating mechanism for vestibular inputs would result in difficulties in maintaining balance. Indeed, this is a classic feature of lesions of the flocculonodular lobe but is not associated with lesions in the hemispheres of the posterior lobe, anterior limb of the internal capsule, or the dentate nucleus, which are functionally linked to the frontal lobe. Lesions of the anterior lobe also do not affect mechanisms of balance.

3-39. The answer is d. (*Sierles, pp 9–11.*) A depressed mood and depressive illnesses are the most common psychosocial reactions of persons with AIDS. A depressive illness can be secondary to a viral infection of the brain and nervous system or a side effect of drugs used to treat AIDS, or it can arise from preexisting mood disorders. Depressed mood and depressive illnesses can also occur from psychosocial stress generated from such factors as reception of a fatal diagnosis, loss of confidentiality, stigma of having AIDS, rejection by friends and family, loss of independence, loss of bowel and bladder control, or loss of occupational competence. Adaptation is a psychosocial factor that affects depression, especially in terms of what the illness means to the patient—e.g., the illness as a challenge, an enemy, a punishment, a weakness, a strategy for life, an irreparable loss or injury, an incentive to change behavior, or a threat to coping capacities. Some of the behaviors that can be observed in depressed moods and illnesses include a sad, apathetic, or anxious mood, loss of self-esteem, guilt, hopeless or helpless feelings, insomnia, loss of appetite, and suicidal thoughts.

3-40. The answer is d. *(Cotran, 5/e, pp 178–190.)* The reaction in the question is a type 2 hypersensitivity reaction that is mediated by antibodies reacting against antigens present on the surface of cells, in this case blood group antigens or irregular antigens present on the donor's red blood cells. Type 2 hypersensitivity reactions result from attachment of antibodies to changed cell surface antigens or to normal cell surface antigens. Complement-mediated cytotoxicity occurs when IgM or IgG binds to a cell surface antigen with complement activation and consequent cell membrane damage or lysis. Blood transfusion reactions and autoimmune hemolytic anemia are examples of this form. Systemic anaphylaxis is a type 1 hypersensitivity reaction in which mast cells or basophils that are bound to IgE antibodies are reexposed to an allergen, which leads to a release of vasoactive amines that cause edema and broncho- and vasoconstriction. Sudden death can occur. Systemic immune complex reactions are found in type 3 reactions and are due to circulating antibodies that form complexes upon reexposure to an antigen, such as foreign serum, which then activates complement followed by chemotaxis and aggregation of neutrophils leading to release of lysosomal enzymes and eventual necrosis of tissue and cells. Serum sickness and Arthus' reactions are examples of this. Delayed-type hypersensitivity is type 4 and is due to previously sensitized T lymphocytes, which release lymphokines upon reexposure to the antigen. This takes time—perhaps up to several days following exposure. The tuberculin reaction is the best known example of this. T-cell-mediated cytotoxicity leads to lysis of cells by cytotoxic T cells in response to tumor cells, allogenic tissue, and virus-infected cells. These cells have CD8 antigens on their surfaces.

3-41. The answer is e. *(April, 3/e, p 613.)* The patient has facial paralysis, which indicates injury to the facial nerve. A problem in the internal auditory meatus usually affects hearing and balance. That the superior salivatory nucleus is normal is indicated by normal lacrimation. Hence, the lesion must be distal to the origin of the greater superficial nerve at the genu of the facial nerve. However, absence of hyperacusis indicates that the branch to the stapedius muscle is functioning normally, and this fact suggests that the lesion is close to the stylomastoid foramen. Loss of taste and diminished salivation locate the lesion proximal to the origin of the chorda tympani nerve. If the lesion were distal to the stylomastoid foramen, taste and salivation would have been normal with facial paralysis as the only sign.

3-42. The answer is a. *(Fauci, 14/e, p 1982.)* Transsphenoidal surgery has the advantages of potential cure with rapid therapeutic response. If the tumor is completely resected, the patient may experience a complete cure. Medical therapy with somatostatin agonist or bromocryptine is helpful, but the patient is dependent on medical therapy indefinitely. Irradiation takes years for full effectiveness, and the patient may develop hypopituitarism. Transfrontal surgery is rarely employed now.

3-43. The answer is c. *(Hardman and Limbird, 9/e, pp 415–416.)* NMS is thought to be a severe form of an extrapyramidal syndrome that can occur at any time with any dose of a neuroleptic agent. However, the risk is higher when high-potency agents are used in high doses, especially if given parenterally. Mortality from NMS is greater than 10%.

3-44. The answer is a. *(Cotran, 5/e, pp 1039–1043.)* Several pathologic conditions are associated with the formation of white plaques on the vulva, which clinically are referred to as leukoplakia. Lichen sclerosus is seen histologically as atrophy of the epidermis with underlying dermal fibrosis. This abnormality is seen in post-menopausal women who develop pruritic white plaques of the vulva. This abnormality is not thought to be premalignant. Loss of pigment in the epidermis, called vitiligo, can also produce leukoplakia. Inflammatory skin diseases, such as chronic dermal inflammation, squamous hyperplasia (characterized by epithelial hyperplasia and hyperkeratosis), and vulvar intraepithelial neoplasia (characterized by epithelial atypia or dysplasia) can also present with leukoplakia. A term related to leukoplakia is vulvar dystrophy, but this term refers specifically to either lichen sclerosis or squamous hyperplasia. Because the latter is sometimes associated with epithelial dysplasia, it is also referred to as hyperplastic dystrophy. It is most commonly seen in postmenopausal women. The male counterpart for lichen sclerosis, which is found on the penis, is called balanitis xerotica obliterans.

Paget's disease is a malignant tumor that can be found in the breast or the vulva. The latter is seen clinically as pruritic red crusted, sharply demarcated map-like areas. Histologically these malignant lesions reveal single anaplastic tumor cells surrounded by clear spaces ("halos") infiltrating the epidermis. These malignant cells stain positively with PAS and mucicarmine stains.

3-45. The answer is d. (*Fauci, 14/e, p 1986.*) This patient's presentation suggests ectopic ACTH secretion, and an ACTH will likely be elevated above 300. An MRI of the pituitary and CT of the abdomen are not useful, since the source of ACTH is from the small cell carcinoma in the lung mass.

3-46. The answer is a. (*Cotran, 5/e, pp 1093–1097.*) Fibrocystic change of the breast is one of the most common features seen in the female breast. It is most likely associated with an endocrine imbalance that causes an abnormality of the normal monthly cyclic events within the breast. These fibrocystic changes are subdivided into nonproliferative and proliferative changes. Nonproliferative changes include fibrosis of the stroma and cystic dilatation of the terminal ducts, which when large may form blue-domed cysts. A common feature of the ducts in nonproliferative changes is apocrine metaplasia, which refers to epithelial cells with abundant eosinophilic cytoplasm with apical snouts. Proliferative changes include epithelial hyperplasia of the ducts. This hyperplastic epithelium may form papillary structures (papillomatosis when pronounced), or may be quite abnormal (atypical hyperplasia). Two benign, but clinically important, forms of proliferative fibrocystic change include sclerosing adenosis and radial scar. Both of these may be mistaken histologically for infiltrating ductal carcinoma, but the presence of myoepithelial cells is a helpful sign that points to the benign nature of the proliferation. Sclerosing adenosis is a disease of the terminal lobules that is typically seen in patients 35 to 45 years old. It produces a firm mass, most often located in the upper outer quadrant. Microscopically there is florid proliferation of small ductal structures in a fibrous stroma, which on low power is stellate in appearance and somewhat maintains the normal lobular architecture. A radial scar refers to ductal proliferation around a central fibrotic area.

3-47. The answer is b. *(Rowland, 9/e, pp 294–302.)* This case is an example of a condition called "normal pressure hydrocephalus." This may be caused by various nonprogressive meningeal and ependymal diseases such as chronic meningitis and subarachnoid hemorrhages, which can initially block CSF absorption. Initially the CSF pressure is high, which results in the enlargement of the ventricles. The CSF pressure becomes normal because the CSF absorption begins again. However, the enlarged ventricles, despite normal CSF pressure, cause hydrostatic impairment to the central white matter surrounding the ventricles. Maximal ventricular expansion is usually located in the frontal lobes with preservation of the cortical gray matter and other subcortical structures. As a result, patients with this condition have diminished frontal lobe functions, namely gait problems without any weakness, as well as urinary incontinence and dementia. Frontal lobe dysfunction can also cause the reappearance of primitive reflexes that disappear shortly after birth, such as the grasp reflex. Late in the course of normal pressure hydrocephalus, the patient may develop "frontal lobe incontinence," where he or she becomes indifferent to the incontinence, much like a very small child. Headaches are rare in this particular type of hydrocephalus. Normal pressure hydrocephalus is usually diagnosed with a thorough neurological examination, in addition to a head CT (computed tomography), which shows enlarged ventricles and occasionally interstitial fluid within the white matter adjacent to the lateral ventricles. Measurement of CSF pressures with a lumbar puncture, and radionuclide cisternography (a procedure where a radionuclide is injected intrathecally, and its distribution is observed over a period of 24 hours) are also helpful. Occasionally, shunting procedures that allow the CSF to drain into the peritoneal cavity or the blood are helpful if performed early in the course of this condition.

3-48. The answer is c. *(Rowland, 9/e, pp 294–302.)* The major mechanism underlying hydrocephalus is decreased absorption of CSF. In the case of normal pressure hydrocephalus, the problem is described above (see answer for the previous question). Another cause of decreased absorption is obstruction of CSF flow by a tumor. Low blood pressure does not cause enlarged ventricles. High blood pressure only causes hydrocephalus as a result of hypertensive crisis, but not chronically. Decreased blood flow in the brain can actually be used as a temporizing measure to acutely decrease intracranial pressure in emergencies, in order to make room for expanding tissue through the mechanism of decreasing pCO_2 in the brain with a ventilator.

3-49. The answer is c. *(Rowland, 9/e, pp 294–302.)* The major location for reabsorption of CSF is the arachnoid villi within the ventricular system. In the case of this particular patient, there is a history of a subarachnoid hemorrhage, which may have caused obstruction within this area.

3-50. The answer is e. *(Rowland, 9/e, pp 294–302.)* The frontal horns of the lateral ventricles are the area of greatest expansion; thus the expansion would affect the adjoining white matter of the frontal lobe. The other areas listed are subcortical and gray matter areas, which are located further from the expanding frontal horns, and less affected. The pituitary gland is quite distant from the frontal horns as well.

BLOCK 4

Answers

4-1. The answer is a. (*Howard, 2/e, pp 479–480.*) Coccidian-like bodies have been identified in stools of some patients with diarrhea. These organisms appear to be similar to blue-green algae and were referred to as *Cyanobacterium*-like until they were recently reclassified as *Cyclospora*. They are larger than the microsporidia and resemble neither *Giardia* nor *Prototheca* nor other algae-like organisms. Unlike *Cryptosporidium*, these organisms fluoresce under ultraviolet light.

4-2. The answer is a. (*Hardman and Limbird, 9/e, p 1146.*) The "red man" syndrome is associated with vancomycin, thought to be caused by histamine release. Prevention consists of a slower infusion rate and pretreatment with antihistamines.

4-3. The answer is b. (*Cotran, 5/e, pp 245–252. Chandrasoma, 3/e, pp 260–264.*) Several gross and microscopic features help to differentiate benign neoplasms from malignant neoplasms. Benign neoplasms grow slowly with an expansile growth pattern that often forms a fibrous capsule. This histologic feature can also be useful in distinguishing a benign neoplastic lipoma from normal non-neoplastic adipose tissue. Benign neoplasms characteristically remain localized and do not metastasize. Histologically benign neoplastic cells tend to be uniform and well-differentiated, that is, they appear similar to their tissue of origin. This histologic feature may not distinguish between benign neoplasms and normal tissue. In contrast to benign tumors, malignant neoplasms grow rapidly in a "crab-like" pattern and are capable of metastasizing. Histologically, the malignant cells are pleomorphic because they differ from one another in size and shape. These cells have hyperchromatic nuclei and an increased nuclear to cytoplasmic ratio. Malignant cells tend to have nucleoli, and mitoses may be frequent. These two features only indicate rapidly proliferating cells and can also be seen in reactive or reparative processes. The mitoses in malignancies, however, tend to be atypical, such as tripolar mitoses. Malignant tumors are graded by their degree of differentiation into well-differentiated, moderately differentiated, and poorly differentiated malignancies. Marked pleomorphism is described as anaplasia. This histologic feature is usually seen in poorly differentiated or undifferentiated malignancies.

4-4. The answer is a. (*Cotran, 5/e, pp 527–528.*) One of the consequences of myocardial ischemia is chest pain, which is called angina. Angina is caused by a mismatch between the myocardial oxygen demand and the myocardial blood flow. There are three main types of angina. Typical angina (stable angina) is the most common type and is characterized by pain that results from exercise, stress, or excitement. The pain is promptly relieved by rest, which decreases oxygen demand, or nitroglycerin. This chemical is converted to nitric oxide, which is a vasodilator that increases perfusion to the heart. EKG changes in patients with stable angina are nonspecific and include T wave inversion and ST segment depression, which occurs secondary to ischemia of the subendocardium of the left ventricle. Prinzmetal angina (atypical angina) is caused by coronary artery vasospasm and is characterized by pain occurring at rest. This pain may be relieved by calcium channel blockers or nitroglycerin. The EKG in these patients reveals ST segment elevation, which is the result of transmural ischemia. The third type of angina is unstable angina, which is characterized by increasing frequency of pain, increased duration of the pain, or pain that is produced by less physical exertion. This final type of angina indicates that a myocardial infarction (MI) may be near, most likely due to the formation of a thrombus over an area of coronary artery atherosclerosis. In contrast to an MI, with angina there is no actual necrosis (infarction) of myocardial tissue, and therefore there are no increased cardiac enzymes, such as LDH and CPK, in the serum. Also, the pain of angina is not made worse with deep inspiration, a sign that is suggestive of pleural disease.

4-5. The answer is a. (*Cotran, 5/e, pp 675–676.*) Atelectasis refers to lung collapse. It is divided into four types. Absorptive (obstructive) atelectasis results from airway obstruction, such as occurs with mucus, tumors, or foreign bodies. The air within the lungs distal to the obstruction is absorbed, the lung collapses, and the mediastinum then shifts toward the collapsed lung. With compression, atelectasis fluid within the pleural cavity, such as seen with congestive heart failure (CHF), causes increased pleural pressure, which collapses lung tissue. In this instance the mediastinum shifts away from the collapsed lung. In contraction atelectasis fibrosis causes collapse of lung tissue. Patchy atelectasis may result from loss of pulmonary surfactant, which is seen in hyaline membrane disease of the newborn.

4-6. The answer is d. *(Cotran, 5/e, pp 1035–1037, 1053–1054.)* The endometrium and myometrium are relatively resistant to infections. Therefore, inflammation of the endometrium (endometritis) is rare. The diagnosis of endometritis depends on finding inflammatory cells within the endometrium that are not present during the normal menstrual cycle. Polymorphonuclear leukocytes (neutrophils) are normally present during menstruation, while a stromal lymphocytic infiltrate can be seen at other times during the menstrual cycle. Lymphoid aggregates and lymphoid follicles may also be seen in normal endometrium. Therefore the presence of any of these types of leukocytes is not diagnostic of endometritis. Acute endometritis is usually caused by bacterial infections following delivery or a miscarriage and is characterized by the presence of neutrophils in endometrial tissue that is not menstrual endometrium. The histologic diagnosis of chronic endometritis depends on finding plasma cells within the endometrium. All it takes is one plasma cell to make the diagnosis. Chronic endometritis may be seen in patients with intrauterine devices (IUDs), pelvic inflammatory disease (PID), retained products of conception (postpartum), or tuberculosis. The latter is characterized histologically by the presence of caseating granulomas with Langhans giant cells. These are secondary causes of chronic endometritis. In a significant number of cases, no underlying cause is found. Decidualized stromal cells are the result of the effects of progesterone and are seen normally in the late secretory phase or in patients who are pregnant. Histologically these stromal cells have abundant eosinophilic cytoplasm.

4-7. The answer is c. *(Kandel, 3/e, pp 654–656.)* Sam has Parkinson's disease, a degenerative condition caused by progressive loss of dopaminergic cells in the substantia nigra pars compacta. This is an area that controls the speed and spontaneity of movement, so damage to this area can produce deficits that include: a slow, shuffling gait with a tendency to move progressively faster ("festinating" gait), problems with maintaining size in handwriting, with a tendency to write with small letters (micrographia), mask-like facial expression with a paucity of eye-blinks, and difficulty getting out of a chair. Other problems include a soft, monotonous voice, muscle rigidity (lead-pipe rigidity), a tremor at rest which is "pill-rolling," and a combination of a tremor and rigidity, especially in the arms, which, when flexion is attempted, elicits a "cogwheeling" property. Failure to swallow with a normal frequency makes drooling a problem. Dementia (senility) is also a problem with Parkinson's patients, especially later in the course of the disease.

4-8. The answer is d. (*Kandel, 3/e, p 1042.*) The blood supply to the substantia nigra arises from the posterior circulation, specifically the posteromedial branches of the posterior cerebral artery and branches of the posterior communicating artery. The lenticulostriate branches of the middle cerebral artery supply other portions of the basal ganglia, such as the striatum and the globus pallidus. The anterior choroidal artery also supplies some of the telencephalic nuclei of the basal ganglia.

4-9. The answer is c. (*Kandel, 3/e, pp 654–656.*) The majority of cells that are lost in this disease are dopaminergic cells in the substantia nigra, pars compacta. Only the pars compacta region of the substantia nigra contains dopaminergic neurons.

4-10. The answer is e. (*Kandel, 3/e, p 655.*) Medications are currently available to lessen the symptoms of Parkinson's disease. Some of these medications contain various concentrations of L-dopa, an immediate precursor to dopamine. Dopamine itself doesn't cross the blood-brain barrier, so it cannot be directly replaced.

4-11. The answer is b. (*Fauci, 14/e, p 1994.*) This patient has a classic history for hypopituitarism. During surgical stress, she will require an increased replacement dose of steroids. The other treatments will not cover her need for increased glucocorticoids and will not be helpful.

4-12. The answer is b. (*Sierles, pp 76–80.*) Contingency management is the technical term often used for positive reinforcement or stepping. It involves the process of changing the frequency of a behavior by controlling the consequences of that behavior with positive reinforcement to encourage or discourage a particular behavior. The procedure is used daily in our family and professional lives, such as rewarding (or punishing) a child for his behavior and receiving (or being denied) a raise at work. Thus, a particular behavior becomes associated with a certain positive or negative consequence and the individual eventually accepts the desired behavior as being preferable. Behavior therapists have developed a wide range of applications for this learning procedure. A successful example is the "token economy" program (receiving tokens redeemable for snacks, movies, special privileges, etc.), which rewards destructive individuals for exhibiting appropriate behavior such as participating in rehabilitation activities. Contingency management has been effective with chronically hospitalized schizophrenic patients, such as the patient in the question who was disrupting the ward by shouting in the hall. Often, well-timed praise or friendliness will serve as an appropriate reinforcer to foster patient compliance, as will a lollipop for a child, or a follow-up phone call to a patient who has recovered or stopped smoking to reinforce your interest in their wellness, as well as their illness.

In stimulus control, the attempt is to eliminate the stimulus or cue that triggers undesired behavior. Modeling exposes the individual to desirable behavior or stimuli (e.g., posters or advertisements showing high status persons resisting smoking or explaining how to resist peer pressure).

4-13. The answer is e. *(Cotran, 5/e, p 1121.)* The syndrome of inappropriate antidiuretic hormone (SIADH) is an important cause of dilutional hyponatremia that has been identified in tumors of the thymus gland, malignant lymphoma, and pancreatic neoplasms. It occurs predominantly, however, as a result of ectopic secretion of ADH by oat cell carcinomas of the lung. Since the tumor cells per se are autonomously producing ADH, there is no feedback inhibition from the hypothalamic osmoreceptors, and the persistent ADH effect on the renal tubules causes water retention even with concentrated urine. Hence the term inappropriate ADH arises. Laboratory findings of the syndrome include low plasma sodium levels (dilutional hyponatremia), low plasma osmolality, and high urine osmolality caused by disproportionate solute excretion without water.

4-14. The answer is b. *(Rhoades, pp 380–383, 395–398.)* Under normal conditions the $\dot{V}/\dot{Q}$ ratio in both lungs is the same, so that mixed alveolar gas in both lungs have the same P_{O_2} and P_{CO_2}. The gas from the normal lung will be approximately normal (P_{O_2} = 100 mmHg, P_{CO_2} = 40 mmHg). While the gas from the occluded lung, which now represents alveolar dead space, will resemble tracheal gas (P_{O_2} = 150 mmHg, P_{CO_2} = 0 mmHg). When the gas from the two lungs mix, the average alveolar O_2 becomes 125 mmHg and the average P_{CO_2} becomes 20 mmHg.

4-15. The answer is b. (*Alberts, 3/e, pp 734–749. Cotran, 5/e, pp 37–39.*) Many extracellular substances cause intracellular actions via second messenger systems. These second messengers may bind to receptors that are located either on the surface of the cell or within the cell itself. Substances that react with intracellular receptors are lipid soluble (lipophilic) molecules that can pass through the lipid plasma membrane. Examples of these lipophilic substances include thyroid hormones, steroid hormones, and the fat soluble vitamins A and D. Once inside the cell these substances generally travel to the nucleus and bind to the hormone response element (HRE) of DNA.

Some substances that react with cell surface receptors bind to guanine-nucleotide regulatory proteins. These proteins, called G proteins, may be classified into four categories, namely Gs, Gi, Gt, and Gq. Two of these receptors, Gs and Gi, regulate the intracellular concentration of cyclic adenosine 5'- monophosphate (cAMP). In contrast, Gt regulates the intra-cytoplasmic levels of cyclic guanosine 5'-monophosphate (cGMP), and Gq regulates the intracytoplasmic levels of calcium ions. Gs and Gi regulate intracellular cAMP levels by their actions on adenyl cyclase, an enzyme located on the inner surface of the plasma membrane that catalyzes the formation of cAMP from ATP. The adenylate cyclase G protein complex is composed of the following components: the receptor, the catalytic enzyme (i.e., adenyl cyclase), and a coupling unit. The coupling unit consists of GTP-dependent regulatory proteins (G-proteins), which may either be stimulatory (Gs) or inhibitory (Gi). These G-proteins consist of three fragments: the α unit (either αs or αi), the β unit, and the γ unit. The α units are active only when complexed to GTP (Gαs-GTP and Gαi-GTP), and they are inactivated when GTP is converted to GDP, which forms Gαs-$\beta\gamma$ and Gαi-$\beta\gamma$. To summarize, when bound to GTP and active, Gs stimulates adenyl cyclase and increases cAMP levels. (Gs can be thought of as the "on switch.") In contrast, when bound to GTP and active, Gi inhibits adenyl cyclase and decreases cAMP levels. (Gi can be thought of as the "off switch.") It is important to note that cholera toxin and pertussis toxin both act by altering this adenyl cyclase pathway. Cholera toxin inhibits the conversion of Gs-GTP to Gs-GDP. In contrast, pertussis toxin inhibits the activation of Gi-GDP to Gαi-GTP. Therefore, both cholera toxin and pertussis toxin prolong the functioning of adenyl cyclase and therefore increase intracellular cAMP, but their mechanisms are different. Cholera toxin keeps the "on switch" in the "on" position, while pertussis toxin keeps the "off switch" in the "off" position.

4-16. The answer is e. *(Cotran, 5/e, pp 1300–1304.)* Neural tube developmental defects are caused by defective closure of the neural tube. These defects, which may occur anywhere along the extent of the neural tube, are associated with maternal obesity and decreased folate during pregnancy. Neural tube defects are associated with increased maternal serum levels of alpha fetoprotein (AFP), which is a glycoprotein synthesized by the yolk sac and the fetal liver. Increased serum levels are also associated with yolk sac tumors of the testes and liver cell carcinomas. Neural tube defects are classified based on their location into caudal or cranial defects. Failure of development of the cranial end of the neural tube results in anencephaly. This abnormality, which is not compatible with life, is characterized by the absence of the forebrain. Instead there is a mass of vascularized neural tissue in this area, which is called the cerebrovasculosa.

Spina bifida is a general term that refers to abnormal fusion of the vertebral arches of the lowest vertebral arches, usually the sacrolumbar region. There are several disorders in this group of developmental abnormalities that have varying degrees of severity. Spina bifida occulta is the mildest form and is characterized by failure of vertebral fusion only. The spinal cord and meninges are normal. In spina bifida occulta the defect in the closure of the neural tube is covered by skin and dermis, with only a pinpoint sinus or hair-covered depression marking the site. Bacterial meningitis, or meningomyelitis, is the major potential risk in these patients. The remaining types of spina bifida are classified as spina bifida cystica. Spina bifida with a meningocele is characterized by protrusion of a meningeal sac filled with cerebrospinal fluid (CSF) through the vertebral defect. Because the cord is in its normal location, there are minimal neurologic deficits. Next in severity is spina bifida with a myelomeningocele, which is characterized by herniation of the cord and a meningeal sac through the vertebral defect. This abnormality is often associated with severe neurologic defects in the lower extremities, bladder, and rectum. The most severe form of spina bifida, spina bifida aperta or myeloschisis, results from complete failure of fusion of the caudal end of the neural plate, which lies open on the skin surface. This abnormality also results in severe neurologic defects in the legs, bladder, and rectum.

Cranium bifidum refers to ossification defects of the occipital bone. The abnormalities produced by these defects are somewhat analogous to spina bifida. There may be protrusion of meninges (cranial meningocele), meninges and brain (meningoencephalocele), or meninges, brain, and ventricles (meningohydroencephalocele). Meningoencephalocystocele (a herniation at the roof of the mouth) together with cranial meningocele and cranial meningoencephalocele occur less frequently than the herniations associated with spina bifida. Cerebral palsy refers to any nonheritable, nonprogressive neurologic motor deficit with onset during the perinatal period, regardless of the etiology. Two examples of cerebral palsy are spastic diplegia and infantile hemiplegia. Spastic diplegia is characterized by spastic weakness of all four extremities, while infantile hemiplegia, usually resulting from unilateral infection or thrombosis of cerebral vessels, is associated with mild mental retardation and convulsions.

4-17. The answer is d. (*Cotran, 5/e, pp 879–882. Chandrasoma, 3/e, pp 659–662.*) The most common primary malignancy of the liver is the hepat-ocellular carcinoma (hepatoma). These tumors are associated with certain viral infections (hepatitis B and hepatitis C viruses), aflatoxin (produced by *Aspergillus flavus*), and cirrhosis. Microscopic sections of these tumors reveal pleomorphic tumor cells that form trabecular patterns, which are similar to the normal architecture of the liver. Hepatomas may secrete α-fetoprotein (AFP), but this tumor marker may also be seen in yolk-sac tumors or fetal neural tube defects. Clinically hepatocellular carcinomas have a tendency to grow into the portal vein or the inferior vena cava, and may be associated with several types of paraneoplastic syndromes, such as polycythemia, hypoglycemia, and hypercalcemia. There is a microscopic fibrolamellar variant of hepatocellular carcinoma that is seen more often in females, is not associated with AFP, is grossly encapsulated, and has a better prognosis. It is important to compare the characteristics of hepatocellular carcinomas with another type of primary tumor of the liver, namely cholangiocarcinoma, which is a malignancy of bile ducts. This tumor is associated with Thorotrast and infection with the liver fluke (*Clonorchis sinensis*), but it is not associated with cirrhosis. Histologically, the tumor cells have cytoplasmic mucin, which is not found in hepatomas. Instead these malignant cells may have cytoplasmic bile. Malignant metastatic tumors are the most common tumors found in the liver.

Grossly there may be multiple or single nodules, while microscopically they usually resemble the primary tumor. For example, metastatic colon cancer to the liver will histologically reveal adenocarcinoma. Metastatic disease to the liver usually does not cause functional abnormalities of the liver itself, and the liver enzymes and bilirubin levels in the blood are usually normal. Angiosarcomas are highly aggressive malignant tumors that arise from the endothelial cells of the sinusoids of the liver. Their development is associated with certain chemicals, such as vinyl chloride, arsenic, and Thorotrast. A malignant tumor of the liver that is found in children is the hepatoblastoma. Microscopically these tumors consist of ribbons and rosettes of fetal embryonal cells.

4-18. The answer is a. (*McPhee, 2/e, p 7.*) About 50 percent of cases of neurofibromatosis are due to new mutations. Hypermorphism is a mutation that produces an increase in function. A dominant negative mutation gives rise to a protein that interferes with the function of the normal allele. One copy of the dominant negative allele has the same effect as two copies of the allele. This effect is called antimorphic.

4-19. The answer is a. (*Fauci, 14/e, pp 618–619.*)

4-20. The answer is d. (*Cotran, 5/e, pp 158–159.*) The Barr body represents a sex chromatin clump attached to the nuclear membrane that originates from an entire X chromosome and can easily be seen by using light microscopy to examine scrapings of the epithelium of the inside buccal mucosa. According to the formula $M = n - 1$, the total number of X chromatin masses equals the number of cellular X chromatin masses seen in the nucleus minus 1. Hence, normal males are $0 = 1 - 1$ (no Barr body), and normal females are $1 = 2 - 1$ (one Barr body). In classic Turner's syndrome (XO), the expected buccal smear would be $0 = 1 - 1$ (no Barr bodies seen), as in a normal male. Karyotyping is necessary when the Barr body screening test is ambiguous or inconclusive. In a young female of short stature and average intelligence who has never menstruated, there is a strong indication that one of the forms of Turner's syndrome exists, and the presence of one Barr body indicates that the patient has XX in some percentage of cells. About 10 percent of all Turner's syndrome patients show a mosaic pattern, with some cells having XO/XX or XO/XXX patterns. In this example, the patient is likely to be XO/XX by the formula 1 = 2 − 1. In Turner's mosaics, the likelihood of developing a seminoma or gonadoblastoma is higher than expected, and gonadectomy may be indicated.

4-21. The answer is d. *(Hardman and Limbird, 9/e, pp 1247, 1335.)* Leucovorin prevents methotrexate from inhibiting dihydrofolate reductase and reverses all of its adverse effects except neurotoxicity.

4-22. The answer is a. *(April, 3/e, pp 133, 140.)* The deep incisure in the inferior border of the pedicle ensures that the spinal nerve associated with that vertebra will exit through the intervertebral foramen well above the intervertebral disk so that it will not be affected by a herniation at that level. However, a posterolateral herniation (the usual direction) will impinge upon the next lower nerve as it courses toward its associated intervertebral foramen. In this case, pain was distributed along the medial side of the leg and foot as far as the great toe—the distribution of the saphenous branch of the femoral nerve (L4). Herniation of the third lumbar intervertebral disk between vertebral bodies L3-L4 would affect nerve L4.

4-23. The answer is a. *(Fauci, 14/e, p 1975.)* A common presentation for hyperprolactinemia is amenorrhea. Important in the initial evaluation of amenorrhea is a determination of the prolactin level. Estradiol and progesterone typically are not measured in an initial evaluation of amenorrhea. Testosterone and DHEA-S are markers for androgen excess, which may be present in this patient, but do not need to be measured initially.

4-24. The answer is b. *(Fauci, 14/e, pp 1975 and 2131.)* This patient may have multiple endocrine neoplasia syndrome-1, which presents with pituitary tumors, pancreatic tumors, and hyperparathyroidism. With the history of severe peptic ulcer disease (possible Zollinger-Ellison syndrome) and family history of pituitary tumors, one must suspect MEN-1. A serum calcium determination will be useful in diagnosing potential hyperparathyroidism. Elevated calcitonin and urinary metanephrine levels are characteristic of MEN-2. Serum ferritin and fasting blood sugar levels would be elevated in hemochromatosis.

4-25. The answer is d. *(Kandel, 3/e, p 729.)* This is an example of the "locked-in syndrome," or pseudocoma, caused by an infarction of the pontine tegmentum. Because the tracts mediating movement of the limbs and face run through this region, the patient is unable to move the face, as well as both arms and legs. Consciousness and eye movements are preserved.

4-26. The answer is c. *(Kandel, 3/e, p 729.)* The pontine tegmentum is mainly supplied by the basilar artery. Complete occlusion of this artery causes deficits on both sides, since this artery supplies both sides of the pons.

4-27. The answer is a. *(Kandel, 3/e, p 729.)* Basilar artery occlusion causes damage to the basilar pons, where the corticospinal and corticobulbar tracts run. These tracts contain motor fibers mediating movement of the limb and face, respectively. This results in complete paralysis to both sides of the body and the face. None of the tracts in the other choices mediate conscious movement.

4-28. The answer is e. *(Adams, 6/e, p 805.)* Sensory loss, including loss of proprioception (feeling the movement of a limb) also occurs as a result of damage to the medial lemniscus bilaterally. This tract contains fibers from the dorsal columns, and also runs through the pontine tegmentum.

4-29. The answer is d. *(Cotran, 5/e, pp 411–414.)* The symptoms of vita-min A deficiency result from abnormalities involving the normal functions of vitamin A. These normal functions include maintaining mucus-secreting epithelium, restoring levels of the visual pigment rhodopsin, increasing immunity to infections, and acting as an antioxidant. Deficiencies of vita-min A will result in squamous metaplasia of mucus membranes, not intesti-nal metaplasia. Squamous metaplasia of the respiratory tract will lead to increased numbers of pulmonary infections due to lack of the normal pro-tective muco-ciliary "elevator." Squamous metaplasia of the urinary tract will lead to increased numbers of urinary tract stones, while such metapla-sia in sebaceous and sweat glands of dry skin causes follicular hyperker-atosis and predisposes to acne. There are numerous eye changes produced by a vitamin A deficiency. These changes include dry eyes (xerophthalmia), soft cornea (keratomalacia), and elevated white plaques of keratin debris on the conjunctiva (Bitot's spots). Because vitamin A is important in the nor-mal function of rhodopsin, a visual pigment important for vision in dim light, a deficiency of vitamin A is associated with poor vision in dim light.

This night blindness is usually the first symptom seen in patients with a vitamin A deficiency.

Rather than causing acute leukemia, vitamin A is used with good results in the treatment of a particular type of acute leukemia, namely acute promyelocytic leukemia. Megaloblastic anemia is associated with a deficiency of either vitamin B12 or folate, while a deficiency of vitamin D will lead to decreased mineralization of bones (soft bones).

4-30. The answer is c. (*Chandrasoma, 3/e, pp 799–806.*) Granuloma inguinale is a rare, sexually transmitted disease that is caused by *Calymmatobacterium donovani*, a small, encapsulated gram-negative bacillus. Infection results in a chronic disease that is characterized by superficial ulcers of the genital region. Regional lymph node involvement produces large nodular masses that develop extensive scarring. Specialized culture media is available, but its use is not practical. Serologic tests are also not useful. Instead, histologic examination is used to demonstrate Donovan bodies, which are organisms within the cytoplasm of macrophages. They are seen best with silver stains or Giemsa's stain. Chancroid is an acute venereal disease that is characterized by painful genital ulcers with lymphadenopathy. It is caused by *Hemophilus ducreyi*, a small, gram-negative bacillus. Gram stains of the suppurative lesions or cultures on specialized media may be used to make the diagnosis. Serologic tests are not useful. *Neisseria gonorrhea*, a gram-negative diplococcus, causes gonorrhea, an acute suppurative infection of the genital tract. In males it produces a purulent discharge (urethritis) and dysuria. In women, it may be asymptomatic (50 percent), or it may produce infection of the cervix with a vaginal discharge, dysuria, and abdominal pain. Ascending infections in women can lead to salpingitis, tubo-ovarian abscess, and pelvic inflammatory disease (PID). Fitz-Hugh-Curtis syndrome refers to perihepatitis infection. In newborns, infection acquired during birth can produce a purulent conjunctivitis (ophthalmia neonatorum). This disease has been prevented due to prophylactic therapy to newborn infants. A Gram stain of the urethral or cervical exudate may reveal the intracytoplasmic gram-negative diplococci, or the exudate can be cultured on special media. Serologic tests are not useful. Characteristically, *N. gonorrhea* produces acid from glucose, but not maltose or lactose. The spirochete *Treponema pallidum*, the causative agent of syphilis, has not been grown on any culture media; therefore, other means are available to aid in the diagnosis of syphilis. Dark-field or immunofluorescence examination may be used to detect organisms in the genital ulcers of primary syphilis. Antibodies to cardiolipin, a substance in beef heart that is similar to a lipoid released by *T. pallidum*, are used to screen for syphilis. This is the basis of both the VDRL and the RPR (rapid plasma reagin) tests; however, these screening tests are not totally specific. *Chlamydia* are obligate intracellular parasites that form elementary bodies and reticulate bodies. The former are small, extracellular, and infectious, while the latter are intracellular forms and are noninfectious. Three *Chlamydia* species are *C. psittaci, C. pneumoniae,* and *C. trachomatis*. The last causes several human diseases including trachoma, inclusion conjunctivitis, nongonococcal urethritis, and lymphogranuloma venereum. Specialized culture media and direct examination procedures are available to aid in the diagnosis of these diseases. The regional lymph nodes in patients with lymphogranuloma venereum have a characteristic histologic appearance characterized by necrotizing granulomas forming stellate areas of necrosis. Trachoma is the leading cause of blindness in underdeveloped countries. It is a chronic infection of the conjunctiva that eventually scars the conjunctiva and cornea. Lymphogranuloma venereum (LGV) is a sexually transmitted disease that is characterized by the formation of a genital ulcer with local necrotizing lymphadenitis. The skin test for LGV is the Frei test, which consists of intradermal injection of LGV antigen. Finally, *C. psittaci* is the causative agent of psittacosis (parrot fever). It produces a severe pulmonary disease and should be suspected in patients with a history of bird contact, such as pet shop workers or parrot owners.

4-31. The answer is a. (*Cotran, 5/e, pp 707–708, 715–716.*) Hypersensitivity pneumonitis refers to immunologically mediated interstitial lung diseases that are the result of exposure to specific antigens. Affected individuals have an abnormal sensitivity to the antigen. In contrast to asthma, hypersensitivity pneumonitis primarily involves the alveolus. A classic example of a hypersensitivity pneumonitis is Farmer's lung, which is caused by exposure to thermophilic actinomyces that grows on moldy hay. Byssinosis is a hypersensitivity that is caused by inhalation of cotton, flax, or hemp dust. Prolonged exposure causes chronic lung disease with chronic bronchitis, emphysema, and interstitial granulomas. Two other examples of hypersensitivity pneumonitis include byssinosis (caused by exposure to cotton), and Bird-breeder's lung (caused by exposure to bird droppings). Progressive massive fibrosis (PMF) is not a hypersensitivity reaction but is most commonly caused by exposure to coal (coal workers pneumoconioses) or silica.

4-32. The answer is d. (*Baron, 4/e, pp 731–732.*) Respiratory syncytial virus (RSV) is the most important cause of pneumonia and bronchiolitis in infants. The infection is localized to the respiratory tract. The virus can be detected rapidly by immunofluorescence on smears of respiratory epithelium. In older children the infection resembles the common cold. Aerosolized ribavirin is recommended for severely ill hospitalized infants.

4-33. The answer is d. (*Murray, 24/e, pp 126–129. Stryer, 4/e pp 544, 553.*) All of the poisons shown effect either electron transport or oxidative phosphorylation. Dinitrophenol is unique in that it disconnects the ordinarily tight coupling of electron transport and phosphorylation. In its presence, electron transport continues normally with no oxidative phosphorylation occurring. Instead, heat energy is generated. The same principle is utilized in a well-controlled way by brown fat to generated heat in newborn humans and cold-adapted mammals. The biological uncoupler in brown fat is a protein called thermogenin. Barbiturates, the antibiotic piericidin A, the fish poison rotenone, dimercaprol, and cyanide all act by inhibiting the electron transport chain at some point.

4-34. The answer is d. (*Hardman and Limbird, 9/e, p 564.*) A long-acting benzodiazepine, such as diazepam, is effective in blocking the secobarbital withdrawal symptoms. The anxiolytic effects of buspirone take several days to develop, obviating its use for acute severe anxiety.

4-35. The answer is e. (*Cotran, 5/e, pp 1093–1097.*) The spectrum of benign breast disease includes fibrocystic disease, which is probably a misnomer; adenosis, both sclerosing and microglandular; intraductal papillomas and papillomatosis; apocrine metaplasia; fibrous stromal hyperplasia; and hyperplasia of the epithelial cells lining the ducts and ductules of the breasts. At one time or another each of the above was considered to be a forerunner of carcinoma; however, with extensive studies in the literature, none of these has been shown to necessarily correlate with a greater risk of developing carcinoma with the exception of epithelial hyperplasia, particularly when atypical. With any of the features, but especially epithelial hyperplasia, adding a positive family history of breast cancer in a sibling, mother, or maternal aunt markedly increases the risk for developing carcinoma of the breast in the given patient. Owing to the advances and technology of xeromammography, there has been an increased interest in calcifications, which are markers for carcinoma of the breast. These calcifications, however, do not necessarily occur within the cancerous ducts themselves and can be found frequently in either adenosis adjacent to the carcinoma or even in normal breast lobules in the region. Stipple calcification as seen by xeromammography is regarded by some workers as an indication for a biopsy of the region.

4-36. The answer is b. (*Cotran, 5/e, pp 210–213.*) The constellation of Raynaud's phenomenon, acral sclerosis, and fibrotic tightening of the muscles of facial expression should raise the specter of progressive systemic sclerosis (scleroderma), a multisystem disease that involves the cardiovascular, gastrointestinal, cutaneous, musculoskeletal, pulmonary, and renal systems through progressive interstitial fibrosis. Small arterioles in the forenamed systems show obliteration caused by intimal hyperplasia accompanied by progressive interstitial fibrosis. Evidence implicates a lymphocyte overdrive of fibroblasts to produce an excess of rather normal collagen. Eventually, myocardial fibrosis, pulmonary fibrosis, and terminal renal failure ensue. Over half of all patients have dysphagia with solid food caused by the distal esophageal narrowing in the disease.

4-37. The answer is d. (*Cotran, 5/e, pp 630–631.*) Decreased numbers of neutrophils in the peripheral blood, neutropenia, may be due to decreased production of neutrophils in the bone marrow or increased peripheral destruction of neutrophils. Decreased production may be caused by megaloblastic anemia, certain drugs, or stem cell defects, such as aplastic anemia, leukemias, or lymphomas. Drug-induced destruction of neutrophil precursors is the most common cause of peripheral neutropenia. With all of these different causes of decreased neutrophil production, the bone marrow will be hypoplastic and there will be a decrease in the number of granulocytic precursors. Some causes of neutropenia will also cause a decrease in the numbers of platelets and erythrocytes (pancytopenia).

In contrast to decreased production, cases of neutropenia secondary to peripheral destruction causes a hyperplasia of the bone marrow, with an increase in the number of granulocytic precursors. Causes of increased destruction of neutrophils include sequestration in the spleen due to hypersplenism (not splenic atrophy), increased utilization, such as with overwhelming infections, and immunologically mediated destruction (immune destruction). Causes of the immune destruction include Felty's syndrome and certain drug reactions, such as aminopyrine and some sulfonamides. Drugs may cause decreased production or increased destruction of neutrophils. In the latter, antibodies are formed against neutrophils, and then these cells are destroyed peripherally. Felty's syndrome refers to the combination of rheumatoid arthritis, splenomegaly, and neutropenia. A significant number of patients with Felty's syndrome will have a monoclonal proliferation of CD8 large granular lymphocytes, unrelated to drug use.

4-38. The answer is c. (*Cotran, 5/e, pp 1077–1078. Chandrasoma, 3/e, pp 809–811.*) Abruptio placenta refers to premature separation of a normally located placenta. This abnormality produces marked hemorrhage, premature labor, and fetal demise. Factors that predispose an individual to abruptio placenta include certain drug use (cocaine, alcohol, smoking), maternal hypertension, preeclampsia, multiparity, and increasing maternal age. Placenta previa occurs when the placenta implants in the lower uterine segment. This may also result in severe bleeding problems at the time of delivery. Vaginal examination of a patient with this condition could also be dangerous. Placenta accreta refers to the absence of the decidua and the direct attachment of the placenta to the myometrium. There is no plane of separation between the placental villi and the myometrium. It is an important cause of post-partum hemorrhage because the placenta fails to separate from the myometrium at the time of labor. The hemorrhage can be life threatening, and a total hysterectomy is the treatment of choice. In both placenta accreta and placenta previa the villi are histologically normal, and there is no trophoblastic proliferation.

Gestational trophoblastic disease refers to abnormal proliferation of trophoblastic tissue and includes hydatidiform mole, the invasive mole, and the malignant choriocarcinoma. These neoplasms all secrete β human chorionic gonadotropin (β-hCG) and should be suspected clinically whenever the uterus is too large for the estimated gestational age and no fetal movement or heart sounds are present.

4-39. The answer is c. (*McPhee, 2/e, pp 531–539; Fauci, 14/e, pp 2106–2108.*) One of the least recognized causes of infertility in a woman is scarring of the uterus postpartum: Asherman's syndrome. It classically follows curettage of the uterus, such as occurred here. Women with this syndrome are infertile because of an inability to implant. Ovarian failure, hypothyroidism, and prolactinoma are all eliminated because she still has scant regular menses. Endometriosis causes painful menses.

4-40. The answer is c. *(April, 3/e, p 498.)* The large occipital artery passes between the base of the skull and the medial surface of the mastoid process. It is frequently torn in a basal skull fracture, which produces battle's sign, a hematoma behind the ear pathognomonic for this type of fracture. The small posterior auricular artery, protected by the parotid gland, is not in jeopardy from a basicranial fracture. The superficial temporal artery is anterior to the ear. The external jugular vein is separated from the basicranial by considerable soft tissue.

4-41. The answer is c. *(Rowland, 9/e, pp 8–10, 56–58.)* The language problem is an example of Broca's aphasia, a deficit seen with lesions of Broca's area and manifested by defects in the "motor" aspect of speech, leaving the patient's speech halting and nonfluent. People with Broca's aphasia tend to repeat certain phrases, as well as leave out pronouns. Since the language centers are usually located on the dominant side of the brain (the left side for a right-handed person), this lesion must be on the left side of Joe's brain. Wernicke's aphasia is a problem with the sensory aspect of speech, where the patient can speak fluently, but the speech sounds like gibberish. The area of disruption in this type of aphasia is usually in Wernicke's area, a region of the posterior superior temporal lobe. Dysarthria is slurred speech, but makes grammatical sense. Alexia is the inability to read. Pure word deafness is a type of sensory aphasia where language, reading, and writing are only mildly disturbed, but auditory comprehension of words is very abnormal. This arises from lesions of the posterior temporal lobe.

4-42. The answer is e. *(Rowland, 9/e, pp 8–10, 56–58.)* Joe's condition is an example of a left inferior frontal lobe cortical stroke including the region of Broca's area and the left precentral gyrus. The weakness on his right side confirms this, since the left side of the brain controls the right side of the body. The right leg is most likely less involved than the arm because the "leg" area of the precentral gyrus extends onto the medial aspect of the frontal lobe, an area served by a different artery than that serving the "arm" and "face" areas. The internal capsule contains motor fibers traveling to the cortex, but usually does not involve language. The thalamus contains many sensory, motor, and association areas, but only rarely causes language problems. Functions of the pontine reticular formation do not include language. The corpus callosum is a white matter structure which connects the hemispheres. Lesions of the posterior aspect may cause language problems, such as alexia without agraphia (the ability to write, but not to read), but would not cause both an aphasia as well as weakness.

4-43. The answer is d. (*Rowland, 9/e, pp 8–10, 56–58.*) The middle cerebral artery subserves the precentral gyrus, the area which has been damaged. The damage can be more widespread, depending upon which portion of the vessel becomes occluded. The anterior cerebral artery supplies the orbitofrontal cortex, deep limbic structures, as well as the cingulate gyrus. The posterior cerebral artery supplies the thalamus, portions of the temporal lobes, and portions of the midbrain. The anterior inferior cerebellar artery supplies the lateral inferior pons and portions of the cerebellum. Perforating branches of the basilar artery supply medial portions of the brainstem. The irregular heart beat observed in this case is an example of aerial fibrillation, a heart rhythm which is often recognized by being "irregularly irregular." This rhythm can cause strokes by throwing small blood clots or emboli from the heart to the cerebral blood vessels and occluding them.

4-44. The answer is b. (*Rowland, 9/e, pp 8–10, 56–58.*) Joe's forehead doesn't droop like the rest of his face because this region receives innervation from both sides of the cerebral cortex, giving this area a "back-up" in case of damage. This can only occur when the lesion is above the level of the VII nerve, where both sides no longer contribute to the innervation of the face. This type of weakness is called a central VII nerve lesion, because it occurs within the central nervous system. A peripheral VII nerve lesion is a lesion within the VII nerve nucleus, or distal. This type of lesion always involves the forehead in addition to the rest of the face. The XII nerve innervates the tongue, the V nerve innervates sensation of the face, in addition to the muscles of mastication, but not the muscles of facial expression. The oculomotor nerve innervates 4 of the muscles which move the eyes.

4-45. The answer is a. (*McPhee, 2/e, p 523.*) Once the female is pregnant, she needs to maintain a high level of progesterone in her system to sustain the fetus. The corpus luteum, sitting in the ovary, has that role, under the influence of the β-hCG produced by the placenta. If the corpus luteum can not produce enough progesterone to get the pregnancy to week 10, the pregnancy is lost.

4-46. The answer is c. *(Sherris, 3/e, pp 550–555.)* A male patient with the presentation as outlined in question 4-46 (fatigue, weight loss, and lymphadenopathy) must be tested for antibodies to HIV. While other antibody tests may be relevant after the primary diagnosis, they must be considered after HIV is ruled out. Certainly infectious mononucleosis is a possibility, but its occurrence in this age group is not as frequent as HIV. Patients are tested first by an ELISA screening test. If this test is positive (X2) then a confirmatory Western blot is performed. A Western blot separates the immune response into antibody production for specific components of the virus, i.e., envelope, gag, etc. The table, on the following page shows the various bands that could be seen on a widely used Western blot and their identification by specific antigen source. There are at least three schemes for interpreting Western blots. Assuming technical competence in the laboratory, one of the more common reasons for falsely positive ELISAs and Western blots is an influenza vaccination within the past few months. A rare patient may have antibody to the cell line used to grow virus. Unlike Lyme disease, there is no reported cross-reactivity with EBV or HTLV. There appears to be no naturally occurring antibody to retroviruses.

Antigen	Source
gp 160	envelope (env) gene product
gp 120	env fragment
gp 41	transmembrane fragment
gp 31	
gp 51	polymerase (pol) gene product
p 66	
p 24	core protein (gag)
	gp = glycoprotein
	p = protein

4-47. The answer is b. *(Cotran, 5/e, pp 364–365. Rubin, 2/e, pp 442, 449–452.)* Intestinal tapeworm (cestode) infections result from eating improperly prepared meat. *Taenia saginata* is acquired from ingesting contaminated beef, *Taenia solium* is acquired from contaminated pork, and *Diphyllobothrium latum* is obtained from contaminated fish. The life cycles of these tapeworms involve larval stages in animals and worm stages in humans. If the contaminated meat contains the larval forms of these organisms, then they may develop into an adult worm in the intestines of infected humans. These individuals generally remain asymptomatic, except that *D. latum* may cause a vitamin B12 deficiency. A very different disease will result from humans eating the eggs of *T. solium*, which may be found in human feces. In this case, the eggs hatch in larva, which then penetrate the gut wall and disseminate via the blood stream to lodge in different organs. There they encyst and differentiate into cysticerci. Multiple cysticerci in the brain produce a "Swiss cheese" appearance grossly, and microscopically a scolex (the head of the worm) is found with hooklets. This disease is called cysticercosis. Another cestode, *Echinococcus granulosa*, is the cause of hydatid disease in humans. Individuals become infected by eating the tapeworm eggs. Patients are usually sheep herders who get the eggs from their dogs. Larvae released from the eggs disseminate most often to the liver (75 percent), but they may also travel to the lungs or skeletal muscle. They form large, slowly growing, unilocular cysts that contain multiple scolices. *Toxocara* species, such as *Toxocara canis* and *Toxocara cati*, are one cause of visceral larval migrans. This disease is characterized by infection of visceral organs by helminthic larvae. The typical patient is a young child who develops hypereosinophilia and hypergammaglobulinemia. Ocular manifestations of toxocariasis are common, especially the loss of vision in one eye in a child. Note that this disease is different from cutaneous larva migrans, which is caused by the larval forms of the hookworms and *Strongyloides stercoralis*.

4-48. The answer is b. (*Cotran, 5/e, pp 117–121, 619–620, 981.*) A fulminating septic state should always be considered whenever the constellation of fever, deteriorating mental status, skin hemorrhages, and shock develops. Such conditions can be seen in gram-negative rod septicemia caused by any of the coliforms (gram-negative endotoxic shock) or fulminant meningococcemia (Waterhouse-Friderichsen syndrome). However, a form of nonbacterial vasculitis termed thrombotic thrombocytopenic purpura (TTP) is notorious for producing a clinical syndrome very similar to fulminating infective states. It is characterized by arteriole and capillary occlusions by fibrin and platelet microthrombi and is usually unassociated with any of the predisposing states seen in disseminated intravascular coagulopathy (DIC), such as malignancy, infection, retained fetus, and amniotic fluid embolism. Macrocytic hemolytic anemia, variable jaundice, renal failure, skin hemorrhages, and central nervous system dysfunction are all seen in TTP and are related to the fibrin thrombi, which can be demonstrated with skin, bone marrow, and lymph node biopsies. There is less coagulopathy in TTP than is found in DIC, and hemolytic anemia is generally not found in idiopathic or autoimmune thrombocytopenic purpura. The condition of patients with TTP may be improved by plasmapheresis, with 80 percent survival.

4-49. The answer is a. (*Cotran, 5/e, pp 328–334, 790–794, 800, 804.*) The causes of diarrhea are immense and may be broadly classified into multiple categories including secretory diarrhea, osmotic diarrhea, and exudative diarrhea. Both secretory and exudative diarrhea may have infectious causes. Several viruses may cause secretory diarrhea. Rotavirus is a major cause of diarrhea in children between the ages of 6 and 24 months. Clinical symptoms consisting of vomiting and watery (secretory) diarrhea begin about 2 days after exposure. Bacterial enterocolitis may be related to either the production of preformed toxins, such as with *Vibrio cholerae* and enterotoxigenic *E. coli*, which is a major cause of "traveler's diarrhea," or it may be related to bacterial invasion of the colon, as seen with salmonella and shigella. *Entamoeba histolytica* is a cause of amebiasis and is endemic in underdeveloped countries. It characteristically produces flask-shaped ulcers in the colon and may embolize to the liver, where it produces amebic liver abscesses. Lactase deficiency, a cause of osmotic diarrhea, is very rarely a congenital disorder, but much more commonly is an acquired disorder seen in adults that results in malabsorption of milk and milk products. The onset of symptoms from ulcerative colitis are most commonly apparent between the ages of 20 and 25.

4-50. The answer is d. (*Hardman and Limbird, 9/e, p 414.*) Antipsychotic agents, particularly prochlorperazine, are also useful as antiemetic agents, thought to be due to dopamine blockade at the stomach and at the chemo-receptor trigger zone of the medulla.

BLOCK 5

Answers

5-1. The answer is c. (*Kandel, 3/e, p 718.*) Gary has a spinal cord syndrome called Brown-Sequard syndrome, or hemisection of the spinal cord. The lesion is not at the cervical level because motor functions of the upper limbs were considered normal. The examiner can pinpoint the location of the lesion by using the "sensory level" or level at which the loss of pain and temperature begin, by remembering that the lesion affects fibers that have entered the spinal cord 1 to 2 levels below it, and then cross to the contralateral side. Therefore, a loss of sensory function at T_{10} level indicates a lesion at T_8 or T_9 level. A level at which motor deficits begin can be helpful as well, but in lesions of the thoracic spinal cord, muscles innervated by thoracic nerves are difficult to test. The examiner still expects weakness in the lower extremities, and this helps to make the diagnosis. The Brown-Sequard syndrome may occur as a result of different types of tumors or infections of the spinal cord.

5-2. The answer is b. (*Kandel, 3/e, p 718.*) Because one half of the spinal cord is damaged, the dorsal columns are damaged, and the patient will have loss of proprioception and vibration ipsilateral to and below the level of the lesion. The loss must be ipsilateral because fibers mediating this type of sensation cross above the level of the lesion. The fasciculus gracilis carries fibers originating from the sacral, lumbar, and lower thoracic levels, and the fasciculus carries those from the upper thoracic and cervical levels. Lissauer's tract carries pain and temperature fibers via the dorsal root entry zone. The Brown-Sequard syndrome may occur as a result of different types of tumors or infections of the spinal cord.

5-3. The answer is c. (*Kandel, 3/e, p 718.*) The spinothalamic tract carries fibers mediating pain and temperature. The primary pain fibers enter the spinal cord and pass 1 to 2 segments in the zone of Lissauer before making synapse with neurons that form the lateral spinothalamic tract. Fibers of the lateral spinothalamic tract then cross to the contralateral side 1 to 2 segments above or before where the primary afferent fibers have entered the cord. Accordingly, pain and temperature are lost below the lesion on the contralateral side. The cuneate and gracile fasciculi mediate proprioception and vibration, and the corticospinal tract mediates voluntary motor function.

5-4. The answer is c. (*Kandel, 3/e, p 718.*) The corticospinal tract mediates voluntary motor function. The fibers cross in the medullary pyramids; thus lesions below this structure cause ipsilateral weakness. The reflexes are brisk, since in an upper motor neuron lesion there is a loss of inhibition to spinal reflexes. Muscle, dorsal root, and femoral nerve damage are all examples of lesions distal to the spinal cord. A frontal lobe lesion would not cause a sensory or motor level, and would probably cause problems more proximally, such as slurred speech.

5-5. The answer is a. (*McPhee, 2/e, p 9.*) Type I osteogenesis imperfecta is mild. Type II is severe and usually lethal in the perinatal period. Type III is considered progressive and deforming. Type IV is deforming, but with normal scleras.

5-6. The answer is c. (*Henry, 19/e, pp 323–324. Cotran, 5/e, p 1117.*) The constellation of cartilaginous-periosteal soft tissue growth of the distal extremities (acromegaly) and growth of the skull and face bones is characteristic of hypersecretion of growth hormone (GH) from an anterior pituitary adenoma. GH modulates the production of hepatic somatomedin (sulfation factor). Somatomedins are small peptides that act on the target organs after being synthesized under the influence of growth hormone. They have insulin-like properties but are immunologically distinct from insulin. In addition to acral-skeletal expansion, patients with hyperpituitarism of the adult-onset variety (occurring after epiphyseal plate closure) have organomegaly, including increased size of the heart, kidneys, liver, and spleen. Cardiac failure is usually the mechanism of death.

5-7. The answer is d. (*Cotran, 5/e, pp 37–41.*) Growth factors are chemicals that are associated with cell growth. For example, fibroblast growth factor (FGF) can induce the growth and proliferation of fibroblasts. Additionally one type of FGF, basic FGF, is capable of inducing all of the stages of angiogenesis, these four stages being basement membrane and extracellular matrix degradation, endothelial migration, endothelial proliferation, and finally endothelial differentiation. The epidermal growth factor family includes epidermal growth factor (EGF) and transforming growth factor-α (TGF-α). These substances can cause proliferation or many types of epithelial cells and fibroblasts. The EGF receptor is *c-erb B₁*. Platelet derived growth factor (PDGF), which is found in platelets, activated macrophages, endothelial cells, and smooth muscle cells, can cause migration and proliferation of fibroblasts, smooth muscle cells, and monocytes. TGF-β, produced by platelets, endothelial cells, T cells, and macrophages, is associated with fibrosis. In low concentrations it causes the synthesis and secretion of PDGF, but in high concentrations it is growth inhibitory due to inhibition of the expression of PDGF receptors.

5-8. The answer is b. *(Cotran, 5/e, p 297. Chandrasoma, 3/e, pp 307–308.)* It is important to understand the difference between the grading and staging of a tumor. First of all, these terms are applied to malignant neoplasms and not to benign neoplasms. Basically, grading is done histologically, while staging is done clinically. Grading of a malignant tumor is based on the histologic degree of differentiation of the tumor cells and on the number of mitoses that are present. These histologic features are thought to be indicators of the aggressiveness of the malignant neoplasm. Cancers are generally classified as grades I through IV. Lower grades, such as grades I and II, are less aggressive and have a better prognosis, while higher grades, such as grades III and IV, are more aggressive and have a worse prognosis. In contrast to grading, the staging of cancers is based on the size of the primary lesion, the presence of lymph node metastases, and the presence of bloodborne metastases. These characteristics are determined by clinical means. One of the common staging classifications is the TNM classification. The "T" refers to the tumor size, the "N" refers to the presence of lymph node metastases, and the "M" refers to the presence of non-lymph node metastases. The location of the tumor is also important, as the TNM classification uses different staging systems depending upon the location of the primary tumor. Lower stages are smaller, localized, and have a better prognosis, while higher stages are larger, widespread, and have a worse prognosis. Staging has proved to be of greater clinical value than grading.

5-9. The answer is e. *(Cotran, 5/e, pp 358–360. Damjanov, 10/e, pp 866–878.)* Rickettsia are obligate intracellular parasites that infect endothelial cells and produce symptoms as a result of vasculitis and microthrombi formation.

Serologic tests for rickettsia include complement fixation tests and the Weil-Felix agglutination reaction. The basis for the latter test is the fact that the sera of infected patients can agglutinate strains of proteus vulgaris. There are numerous types of rickettsia that produce many different diseases. Examples include Rocky Mountain Spotted Fever (RMSF, caused by *R. rickettsii*), epidemic typhus (caused by *R. prowazekii* and spread by the human body louse pediculus humanus), endemic typhus (caused by *R. typhi* and spread by lice), scrub typhus (caused by *R. tsutsugamushi* and spread by mites), ehrlichiosis, and Q fever (caused by *Coxiella burnetii* and spread not by vectors but by inhalation of aerosols). RMSF is found not only in the Rocky Mountains, but also the southeast and south-central United States. The vector in the Rocky Mountains is the wood tick (*Dermacentor andersoni*), while in the southeast it is the dog tick (*Dermacentor variabilis*) and in the south-central United States, the Lone Star tick. The animal reservoir for RMSF are wild rodents and dogs. The rash of RMSF characteristically begins peripherally and spreads centrally to the trunk and face. The pathology involves infection of blood vessels producing thrombosis. Intracellular bacilli form parallel rows in an end-to-end arrangement ("flotilla at anchor facing the wind"). Patients also develop muscle pain and high fever.

Bartonella infections are also characterized by proliferations of blood vessels. Examples of Bartonella include *Bartonella quintana*, *Bartonella henselae*, and *Bartonella bacilliformis*, the causative agent of Oroya fever. *Bartonella quintana* is spread by the human body louse and is the causative agent of trench fever (seen in the trenches of WWI) and bacillary angiomatosis. This latter term refers to a lesion seen in patients with AIDS consisting of a lobular proliferation of capillaries with abundant leukocytoclastic debris. Finally, *Bartonella henselae* is the causative agent of cat-scratch fever. Histologically this disease is characterized by the formation of stellate microabscesses with necrotizing granulomas.

5-10. The answer is b. (*Cotran, 5/e, pp 541–543. Abenhaim L, N Engl J Med 335(9), 609–616. Connolly HM, N Engl J Med 337(9), 581–588.*) Hypertensive heart disease (HHD) can be divided into systemic HHD and pulmonary HHD. Systemic HHD is the result of systemic hypertension, which causes left ventricular (LV) hypertrophy. There is by definition no other cardiac disease present that could cause LV hypertrophy, such as aortic stenosis. Hypertension is a pressure overload on the heart, and as such it causes concentric LV hypertrophy without dilation. In contrast, eccentric hypertrophy is the result of volume overload on the heart. In systemic HHD the LV is stiff as there is decreased LV compliance. In a patient with uncontrolled hypertension, LV dilation would indicate LV failure. Pulmonary HHD indicates right ventricular hypertrophy that is the result of pulmonary disease. By definition this type of heart disease is called cor pulmonale. Pulmonary diseases that can cause cor pulmonale include diseases of the lung parenchyma, such as chronic obstructive pulmonary disease and interstitial fibrosis, and diseases of the pulmonary vessels, such as multiple pulmonary emboli and pulmonary vascular sclerosis. The latter has been associated with the use of the combination of diet drugs fenfluramine and phentermine. This combination has been referred to as "Fen-Phen."

5-11. The answer is b. *(April, 3/e, p 251.)* An increase in the vertical diameter of the chest is accomplished by the diaphragm. The axis for rib rotation passes through both costovertebral articulations, i.e., that between the head of the rib and the vertebral body as well as that between the tubercle of the rib and the transverse process. The axis of rotation extends anteriorly to pass through the contralateral costochondral junction. Thus, as the ribs rotate outward, the sternum (located between the crossed axis from either side) is raised. Compensatory movement occurs at the sternocostal joints. Movement at the sternomanubrial joint changes the sternal angle.

5-12. The answer is c. *(DiPalma, 4/e, p 390. Hardman and Limbird, 9/e, p 810.)* Digitalis inhibits Na^+/K^+, ATPase and hence decreases myocyte Na pumping, resulting in a relative reduction of Ca expulsion from Na-Ca exchange. The consequent increase in free Ca in the cell causes increased intensity of interaction between actin and myosin filaments and enhanced contractility.

5-13. The answer is b. *(Cotran, 5/e, pp 934–938.)* Cystic diseases of the kidney, which may be congenital, acquired, or inherited diseases, have characteristic gross appearances. In two types of cystic renal disease, the numerous cysts are found in both the cortex and medulla. These two types of polycystic disease of the kidney are the infantile type and the adult type. Adult polycystic kidney disease typically presents in adulthood and has an autosomal dominant inheritance pattern. Histologically the cysts are lined by tubular epithelium, while the stroma between the cysts is normal. Adult polycystic renal disease is associated with liver cysts and berry aneurysms, which may rupture and cause a subarachnoid hemorrhage. About one-half of patients with adult polycystic renal disease eventually develop uremia. Infantile polycystic kidney disease typically presents in newborns, has an autosomal recessive pattern of inheritance, and is associated with hepatic cysts (microhamartomas) and congenital hepatic fibrosis. Grossly these renal cysts have a radial spoke arrangement.

In two types of cystic renal disease, the cysts are limited to the medulla. Medullary sponge kidney is usually asymptomatic, is not familial, and has normal sized kidneys with small cysts in the renal papillae. Medullary cystic disease complex (nephronophthisis) has small sclerotic kidneys with multiple cysts at the corticomedullary junction. Individuals with this abnormality present in the first two decades of life with salt wasting polyuria and progressive renal failure. Most cases are familial and display both recessive and dominant inheritance patterns. Two other types of cysts that are not limited to the medulla are simple cysts and acquired cysts. Simple cortical cysts are single, unilateral cysts found in adults that are benign. Patients are usually asymptomatic, but they may present with microscopic hematuria. Acquired polycystic renal disease is associated with chronic renal dialysis. These kidneys are shrunken and have multiple cysts and an irregular surface.

5-14. The answer is e. (*Cotran, 5/e, pp 623–626.*) Disseminated intravascular coagulation (DIC) is a severe thrombohemorrhagic disorder that results from extensive activation of the coagulation sequence. With DIC there is widespread fibrin deposits in the microcirculation, which leads to hemolysis of the red cells (microangiopathic hemolytic anemia), ischemia, and infarcts in multiple organs. Continued thrombosis leads to consumption of platelets and the coagulation factors, which will subsequently lead to a bleeding disorder. The excessive clotting also activates plasminogen and increases plasmin levels, which will cleave fibrin and increase serum levels of fibrin split products. DIC is never a primary disorder, but instead is always secondary to other diseases that activate either the intrinsic or the extrinsic coagulation system. Activation of the intrinsic pathway results from the release of tissue factor into circulation. Examples include obstetric complications, from the release of placental tissue factor, and cancers, from the release of the cytoplasmic granules of the leukemic cells of acute promyelocytic leukemia or from release of mucin from adenocarcinomas.

Coagulation may also result from the activation of the extrinsic pathway by widespread injury to endothelial cells, such as with the deposition of antigen-antibody complexes (vasculitis) or endotoxic damage by microorganisms.

5-15. The answer is d. (*Cotran, 5/e, pp 722–726.*) Lung cancers are classified according to their histologic appearance. First they are divided into two groups based on the size of the tumor cells, namely small-cell carcinomas and non-small cell carcinomas. Small cell carcinomas, also called "oat cell" carcinoma, have scant amounts of cytoplasm, and their nuclei are small, round, and rarely have nucleoli. These malignancies, which are of neuroendocrine origin and display neurosecretory granules on electron microscopy, may cause a variety of paraneoplastic syndromes, such as from the synthesis and secretion of hormones such as ACTH and serotonin. Other effects not well understood on the neuromuscular system include central encephalopathy and Eaton-Lambert syndrome, a myasthenic syndrome resulting from impaired release of acetylcholine and usually associated with pulmonary oat cell carcinoma. Oat cell carcinomas form 20 to 25 percent of primary lung tumors, occur most frequently in middle-aged or older men, have a strong association with cigarette smoking, and carry a poor prognosis. The non-small cell carcinomas are classified as to the differentiation of the tumor cells. Squamous cell carcinomas are characterized by keratin pearl formation, intracytoplasmic keratin, or the formation of intercellular bridges. Adenocarcinomas are characterized by the formation of glandular structures. They typically are found at the periphery of the lung (peripheral carcinomas) and sometimes may be found in an area of previous scar (scar carcinoma). Non-small cell carcinomas of the lung that do have form glands or squamous differentiation are called undifferentiated large cell carcinomas.

A hamartoma is the most common benign tumor of the lung. It is composed mainly of cartilage arranged in a haphazard fashion. Other benign neoplasms of the lung include fibromas (composed of fibroblasts), hemangiomas (composed of blood vessels), and leiomyomas (composed of smooth muscle).

5-16. The answer is a. (*McPhee, 2/e, pp 432, 436, and 529; Barron, 2/e, pp 74–75.*) This patient has the classic triad of diabetes mellitus—polyuria, polyphagia, and polydipsia—in combination with visual problems, which can be a marker of diabetic retinopathy. Deep venous thrombosis, urinary tract infection, and preeclampsia are all complications of pregnancy, but none present like this.

5-17. The answer is d. (*Howard, 2/e, p 457.*) *Helicobacter pylori* was first recognized as a possible cause of gastritis and peptic ulcer by Marshall and Warren in 1984. This organism is readily isolated from gastric biopsies but not from stomach contents. It is similar to *Campylobacter* species and grows on chocolate agar at 37°C in the same microaerophilic environment suitable for *C. jejuni* (Campy-Pak or anaerobic jar [Gas Pak] without the catalyst). *H. pylori*, however, grows more slowly than *C. jejuni*, requiring 5 to 7 days incubation. *C. jejuni* grows optimally at 42°C, not 37°C as does *H. pylori*.

5-18. The answer is c. (*Fauci, 14/e, p 1975.*) Galactorrhea in young females is often associated with hyperprolactinemia. Estradiol and progesterone can be useful markers of gonadal function but not provide further diagnostic information. Similarly, testosterone and DHEA-S do not provide more diagnostic information.

5-19. The answer is a. (*McPhee, 2/e, pp 461–462 and 525–526; Fauci 14/e, pp 2116–2117.*) Prolactin is the major stimulator of breast-milk production. Overproduction of prolactin leads to galactorrhea. Estrogen, progesterone, thyroxine, and cortisol are all needed for proper breast development but play no role in actual milk production.

5-20. The answer is c. (*Cotran, 5/e, pp 888–891. Chandrasoma, 3/e, pp 663, 665–667.*) Patients with obstruction of the common bile duct present clinically with Charcot's triad, which consists of biliary colic, high fever (secondary to cholangitis), and jaundice. Jaundice secondary to extra-hepatic obstruction is associated with normal hemoglobin levels, normal serum indirect bilirubin levels, and increased levels of direct bilirubin and alkaline phosphatase. Common causes of obstruction of the common bile duct include cancer in the head of the pancreas and obstruction by a gall-stone. Clinically these two can be differentiated using Courvoisier's law, which states that in a patient with obstructive jaundice, the presence of a palpable gallbladder is indicative of obstruction due to a cancer of the head of the pancreas. This is because the obstruction causes the gallbladder to dilate. In contrast, most patients with gallstones have cholecystitis, which is associated with a thickened gallbladder wall. This will prevent the gallbladder from dilating. Therefore, if the obstruction is due to a gallstone the gallbladder will not dilate and will not be palpable. Cholecystitis, inflammation of the gallbladder, may be either an acute or chronic response. In acute cholecystitis, which may be associated with a stone (calculous) or lack a stone (acalculous), there is an acute inflammatory response which consists mainly of neutrophils. Acute cholecystitis usually presents with right upper quadrant pain and may constitute a surgical emergency. Chronic cholecystitis, which is associated with stones in more than 90 percent of cases, has a variable histologic appearance, but findings include a thickened muscular wall, scattered chronic inflammatory cells (lymphocytes), and outpouchings of the mucosa (Rokitansky-Aschoff sinuses).

5-21. The answer is b. (*Cotran, 5/e, pp 1054–1055.*) Endometrial tissue located in abnormal locations is still under the cyclic influence of hormones and may produce menorrhagia, dysmenorrhea, and cyclic pelvic pain. Menorrhagia refers to an increased amount of regular bleeding, while dysmenorrhea refers to severe pain during menstruation. The ectopic endometrial tissue may be located within the myometrium or it may be found outside of the uterus. The former, nests of endometrial stroma within the myometrium, is called adenomyosis. It is thought to result from the abnormal downgrowth of the endometrium into the myometrium. Ectopic endometrial tissue outside of the uterus is called endometriosis and histologically reveals endometrial glands, stroma, and hemosiderin pigment (from the cyclic bleeding). Repeated cyclic bleeding in patients with endometriosis can lead to the formation of cysts that contain areas of new and old hemorrhages. Because they grossly contain blood clots, these cysts have been called "chocolate cysts." Endometriosis is thought to possibly arise from metaplasia of coelomic epithelium into endometrial tissue, or implantation of normal fragments of menstrual endometrium either via the fallopian tubes or via the blood vessels. Other sites of endometriosis include the uterine ligaments (associated with dyspareunia), rectovaginal pouch (associated with pain on defecation and low back pain), fallopian tubes (associated with peritubular adhesions, infertility, and ectopic pregnancies), urinary bladder (associated with hematuria), GI tract (associated with pain, adhesions, bleeding, and obstruction), and vagina (associated with bleeding).

5-22. The answer is e. (*Cotran, 5/e, pp 414–418, 423–425.*) Vitamin C (ascorbic acid) is a water-soluble vitamin that is important in many body functions, such as the synthesis of collagen, osteoid, certain neurotransmitters, and carnitine. In the synthesis of collagen, vitamin C functions as a cofactor for the hydroxylation of proline and lysine and for the formation of the triple helix of tropocollagen. Patients with decreased vitamin C (scurvy) will have abnormal synthesis of connective tissue due to abnormal synthesis of collagen along with abnormal synthesis of osteoid. The former will lead to impaired wound healing. In addition, previous wounds may reopen. Because the synthesis of collagen is abnormal, the blood vessels will be fragile. This will lead to bleeding gums, tooth loss, subperiosteal hemorrhage, and petechial perifollicular skin hemorrhages. Abnormal synthesis of osteoid (unmineralized bone) will lead to decreased amounts of osteoid in the bone and increased calcification of the cartilage. Vitamin C also functions as an antioxidant and is important in neutrophil function and iron absorption in the gut. These functions will also be decreased in patients with scurvy. This syndrome is common in elderly people living on a diet deficient in milk, fruits, and vegetables.

In contrast to scurvy, which is caused by a deficiency of vitamin C, rickets is caused by a deficiency of vitamin D. Ricketts is characterized by a lack of calcium. In this abnormality the osteoblasts in bone continue to synthesize osteoid, but this material is not mineralized. This results in increased amounts of osteoid (unmineralized bone) and decreased mineralized bone. In adults this produces osteomalacia and bone pain. Histologically, the bone osteoid seams are markedly increased in thickness. In children this produces rickets, a disease that is characterized by increased osteoid at normal growth centers of bone. This produces wide epiphyses at the wrists and knees and leads to growth retardation. Beriberi is caused by a deficiency of thiamine, pellagra by a deficiency of niacin, and kwashiorkor by a deficiency of protein.

5-23. The answer is e. (*Hardman and Limbird, 9/e, pp 442–443, 415.*) Tardive dyskinesia is an adverse effect of neuroleptic, not tricyclic, antidepressants.

5-24. The answer is a. (*Rhoades, pp 79–83.*) The portion of the basilar membrane vibrated by a sound depends on the frequency of the sound. High frequency sounds produce a vibration of the basilar membrane at the base of the cochlea (near the oval and round windows); low frequency sounds produce a vibration of the basilar membrane at the apex of the cochlea (near the helicotrema). The modiolus is the bony center of the cochlea from which the basilar membrane emerges, the spiral ganglion contains the cell bodies of the auditory nerve fibers, and the stria vascularis is the vascular bed located on the outer wall of the scala media of the cochlea responsible for endolymph secretion.

5-25. The answer is d. (*Cotran, 5/e, pp 160–162, 1156–1157.*) Sexual ambiguity arises when there is disagreement between the various ways of determining sex. Genetic sex is determined by the presence or absence of a Y chromosome. Gonadal sex is based upon the histologic appearance of the gonads. Ductal sex depends on the presence of derivatives of the müllerian or wolffian ducts. Phenotypic or genital sex is based on the appearance of the external genitalia. True hermaphroditism refers to the presence of both ovarian and testicular tissue. Pseudohermaphroditism is a disagreement between the phenotypic and gonadal sex. A female pseudohermaphrodite has ovaries but external male genitalia, while a male pseudohermaphrodite has testicular tissue, resulting from an XY genital sex karyotype, but female external genitalia. Female pseudohermaphroditism results from excessive exposure to androgens during early gestation; most often this is the result of congenital adrenal hyperplasia. Male pseudohermaphroditism results from defective virilization of the male embryo, most commonly caused by complete androgen insensitivity syndrome, also called testicular feminization. Turner's syndrome, which has a 45,X0 karyotype, is characterized by a female phenotype and bilateral streak ovaries. Mixed gonadal dysgenesis consists of one well-defined testis and a contralateral streak ovary. It is a cause of ambiguous genitalia in the newborn.

5-26. The answer is a. (*Cotran, 5/e, pp 231–233.*) Amyloid is a generic term that describes special properties of any protein having a tertiary structure that produces a β-pleated sheet. Amyloid stains brown with iodine ("starchlike"). Histologically the deposits always begin between or outside of cells. Eventually the amyloid deposits may strangle the cells, leading to atrophy or cell death. The histologic diagnosis of amyloid is based solely on its special staining characteristics. It stains pink with the routine hematoxylin and eosin stain, but with the Congo red stain, amyloid stains dark red and has an apple-green birefringence appearance when viewed under polarized light. There are many different types of proteins that stain as amyloid, and these proteins are associated with a wide variety of diseases. These diseases may be either systemic, such as with immune dyscrasias, reactive diseases, or hemodialysis, or they may be localized, such as with senile or endocrine disorders. Immune dyscrasias, such as multiple myeloma or B cell lymphomas, secrete amyloid light (AL) chains, while reactive systemic diseases secrete amyloid associated protein (AA). This protein is a polypeptide derived from serum amyloid-associated protein, which is produced in the liver. Systemic deposits of AA protein complicates various chronic infections and inflammatory processes, most commonly rheumatoid arthritis, other connective tissue diseases, bronchiectasis, and inflammatory bowel disease. Patients on chronic hemodialysis may develop amyloid deposits consisting of β_2-microglobulin. Patients with senile cardiac disease may develop amyloid deposits in the heart consisting of amyloid transthyretin (ATTR), while patients with senile cerebral disease, such as Alzheimer's disease, may develop amyloid deposits in the brain consisting of β_2-amyloid protein. Do not confuse β_2-amyloid protein with β_2 microglobulin, a component of the MHC class I molecule. Patients with medullary carcinoma of the thyroid, a malignancy of the calcitonin-secreting parafollicular C cells of the thyroid, characteristically have amyloid deposits of procalcitonin within the tumor. Finally, patients with type II diabetes mellitus may have amyloid deposits within pancreatic islets consisting of islet amyloid polypeptide.

5-27. The answer is b. (*Sierles, pp 76–79.*) The smoker is being exposed to an aversive stimulus. The physiologic and psychological trauma is so severe and so aversive that the patient may choose to avoid smoking in the future. This can also be regarded as a form of punishment. In positive punishment, an unpleasant stimulus is applied, such as spanking or other acts that produce pain; in negative punishment, a positive reinforcer is removed (e.g., withdrawing use of the family car or other privileges). While punishment is not as effective in changing behavior as other more positive reinforcers, it can be effective, at least in dangerous situations and for the short term. Punishment during a longer period can produce resentment, it does not demonstrate positive alternative behaviors, and with certain persons (e.g., a child or adult who is seeking attention) it can become a substitute for positive reinforcement (i.e., the attention gained during spanking can sometimes outweigh the pain).

5-28. The answer is e. (*Adams, 6/e, p 799.*) Emma has had a stroke resulting from occlusion of medial branches of the left vertebral artery, presumably secondary to atherosclerosis (i.e., cholesterol deposits within the artery which eventually occlude it). The resulting syndrome is called the *medial medullary syndrome*, because the affected structures are located in the medial portion of the medulla. These structures include: the pyramids, the medial lemniscus, the medial longitudinal fasciculus, and the nucleus of the hypoglossal nerve and its outflow tract. Emma's symptoms result from damage to the above structures, and may have been caused by the same process (atherosclerosis) that resulted in her heart disease.

5-29. The answer is e. *(Adams, 6/e, p 799.)* The weakness of her right side was caused by damage to the medullary pyramid on the left side. Her face was spared because fibers supplying the face exited above the level of infarct. However, a lesion in the corticospinal tract of the cervical spinal cord above C5 could cause arm and leg weakness, and spare the face, because facial fibers exit in the rostral medulla. A lesion in the inferior portion of the precentral gyrus of the left frontal lobe would cause right-sided weakness, but would include the face, because this area is represented more inferiorly than are the extremities.

5-30. The answer is a. *(Adams, 6/e, p 799.)* Her unsteady gait was a result of the weakness of her right side, but may also have been the result of the loss of position and vibration sense on that side from damage to the medial lemniscus (as demonstrated by the inability to identify the position of her toe with her eyes closed, and the inability to feel the vibrations of a tuning fork). Without position sense, walking becomes unsteady because it is necessary to feel the position of one's feet on the floor during normal gait. Damage to both the medial lemniscus and pyramids at this level causes problems on the contralateral side because this lesion is located rostral to the level where both of these fiber bundles cross to the opposite side of the brain. Damage to the descending component of the MLF could only affect head and neck reflexes, but not gait. Gait is also unaffected by pain inputs.

5-31. The answer is b. *(Kandel, 3/e, pp 684–685. Adams, 6/e, p 1383.)* Deviation of the tongue occurs because fibers from the hypoglossal nucleus innervate the genioglossus muscle on the ipsilateral side of the tongue. This muscle normally protrudes the tongue toward the contralateral side. Therefore, if one side is weak, the tongue will deviate toward the side ipsilateral to the lesion when protruded. A lesion in the precentral gyrus causes protrusion of the tongue toward the side contralateral to the lesion because it is rostral to the crossing of fibers into the hypoglossal nucleus.

5-32. The answer is a. (*Cotran, 5/e, pp 1181–1187.*) Keratosis refers to the proliferation of keratinocytes with excess keratin production. Seborrheic keratoses are benign, elevated ("stuck-on") lesions that usually occur in older individuals. Histologically these lesions reveal hyperkeratosis with horn and pseudo-horn cysts formation. The sudden development of large numbers of seborrheic keratoses (Leser-Trelat sign) may develop in association with another malignancy. This association with malignancies may also be seen with the malignant type of acanthosis nigricans, which consists of hyperpigmented areas of skin in the groin and axilla.

Keratoacanthomas (KA) are rapidly growing lesions that microscopically reveal a cup-shaped lesion with a central, keratin-filled crater surrounded by keratinocytes having eosinophilic ("glassy") cytoplasm. Atypia may be present, but these lesions are not considered to be malignant. The histologic appearance can make differentiating keratoacanthomas from squamous cell carcinomas on a histologic basis quite difficult. The clinical history of rapid development within several weeks is very helpful in making the correct diagnosis. Most cases of KA spontaneously resolve over several months. Human papillomavirus (HPV) causes several types of verrucae (warts), which are hyperkeratotic lesions. Verrucae vulgaris histologically reveal hyperkeratosis, papillomatosis, and koilocytosis. The latter term refers to large vacuolated cells with shrunken nuclei. Characteristically present are numerous, enlarged keratohyalin granules. Actinic (solar) keratoses, found on sun-damaged skin, microscopically shows hyperkeratosis, parakeratosis, atypia of the epidermal keratinocytes, and degeneration of the elastic fibers in the dermis. The latter finding is referred to as solar elastosis. Clinically actinic keratoses appear as irregular erythematous brown papules. When the atypia of the intraepidermal keratinocytes is extreme (full-thickness), the lesion is referred to as Bowen's disease. These lesions are in fat carcinomas in situ since there is no invasion into the underlying dermis. If invasion were present, the lesion would be diagnostic of a squamous cell carcinoma.

5-33. The answer is b. (*Cotran, 5/e, pp 589–592, 601–603.*) Glucose-6-phosphate dehydrogenase (G6PD) is an enzyme of the hexose monophosphate shunt pathway that maintains glutathione in a reduced (active) form.

Glutathione normally protects hemoglobin from oxidative injury. If the erythrocytes are deficient in G6PD, as occurs in G6PD deficiency, exposure to oxidant drugs, such as the antimalarial drug primaquine, denatures hemoglobin, which then precipitates with erythrocytes as Heinz bodies. Macrophages within the spleen remove these bodies, producing characteristic "bite" cells. These red cells then become less deformable and are trapped and destroyed within the spleen (extravascular hemolysis). The gene for G6PD is located on the X chromosome and has considerable pleomorphism at this site. Two variants are the A type, which is found in 10 percent of African Americans and is characterized by milder hemolysis of younger red cells, and the Mediterranean type, which is characterized by a more severe hemolysis of red cells of all ages. Hereditary spherocytosis (HS), an autosomal dominant disorder, is characterized by an abnormality of the skeleton of the red cell membrane that makes the erythrocyte spherical, less deformable, and vulnerable to splenic sequestration and destruction (extravascular hemolysis). In HS, there is a defect in the spectrin molecule, which then has less binding to protein 4.1. This disorder can be diagnosed in the laboratory by the osmotic fragility test. Paroxysmal nocturnal hemoglobinuria (PNH), an acquired clonal stem cell disorder, is characterized by abnormal red cells, granulocytes, and platelets. The red cells are abnormally sensitive to the lytic activity of complement due to a deficiency of GPI (glycosyl phosphatidyl inositol) linked proteins, namely decay-accelerating factor (DAF, or CD55), membrane inhibitor of reactive lysis (CD55), or CD59 (a C8 binding protein). Complement is activated by acidosis, such as with exercise or sleep, which can produce a red morning urine. Complications of PNH include the development of frequent thromboses and possibly acute leukemia. Autoimmune hemolytic anemia is caused by anti-red cell antibodies and is diagnosed using the Coombs antiglobulin test. Microangiopathic hemolytic anemia refers to hemolysis of red cells caused by narrowing within the microvasculature and is seen in patients with prosthetic heart valves or those with disseminated intravascular coagulation, thrombotic thrombocytopenic purpura, or hemolytic-uremic syndrome.

5-34. The answer is a. (*Cotran, 5/e, p 1079.*) Ectopic pregnancy is a potentially life-threatening condition if it is not treated by removal before rupture and hemorrhage with fatal exsanguination. The most common location for extrauterine implantation is the fallopian tube (more than 85 percent of cases), with rare implantation in the ovary or abdomen. If the tubal implantation has existed from 1 to 4 weeks, the β-hCG test result is likely to be negative; thus a negative result does not exclude pregnancy. It is always worthwhile to repeat a laboratory test when the result is unexpected. Tubal pregnancy is not uncommon and should always be considered if endometrial samples suggest gestational change without chorionic villi.

5-35. The answer is b. *(Fauci, 14/e, pp 618–622.)*

5-36. The answer is c. *(Fauci, 14/e, p 1988.)* This is the common CT finding and clinical presentation for craniopharyngioma. Empty sella does not usually cause marked enlargement of the sella, and there is no cystic structure with calcification. Pituitary macroadenoma can expand the sella but is not commonly cystic and calcified. Optic glioma and hypothalamic hamartoma are rarely cystic.

5-37. The answer is c. *(Murray, 24/e, pp 224, 233. Stryer, 4/e, pp 607–608.)* The most likely cause of the symptoms observed is carnitine deficiency. Under normal circumstances, long chain fatty acids coming into muscle cells are activated as acyl-coenzyme A and transported as acyl carnitine across the inner mitochondrial membrane into the matrix. A deficiency in carnitine, which is normally synthesized in liver, can be genetic; but it is also observed in preterm babies with liver problems and dialysis patients. Blockage of the transport of long chain fatty acids into mitochondria not only deprives the patient of the energy production, but also disrupts the structure of the muscle cell with the accumulation of lipid droplets. Oral dietary supplementation usually can affect a cure. Deficiencies in the carnitine acyltransferase enzymes I and II can cause similar symptoms.

5-38. The answer is c. *(Hardman and Limbird, 9/e, p 1146.)* Vancomycin is often used to treat antibiotic-associated enterocolitis, especially when caused by *C. difficile*. Clindamycin is also associated with *C. difficile* colitis, but in another way: a higher percentage of patients taking this over other antibiotics develop antibiotic-associated enterocolitis.

5-39. The answer is c. *(Cotran, 5/e, pp 632–633. Chandrasoma, 3/e, pp 433–443.)* Lymph nodes may be enlarged (lymphadenopathy) secondary to reactive processes, which can be either acute or chronic reactions. Acute reaction (acute nonspecific lymphadenitis) can result in focal or generalized lymphadenopathy. Focal lymph node enlargement is usually the result of bacterial infection. Sections from involved lymph nodes will reveal infiltration by neutrophils. In contrast, generalized acute lymphadenopathy is usually the result of viral infections and will usually produce a proliferation of reactive T lymphocytes called T immunoblasts. These reactive T cells tend to have prominent nucleoli and can be easily mistaken for malignant lymphocytes or malignant Hodgkin cells.

Reactive processes involving lymph nodes typically involve different and specific portions of the lymph nodes depending upon the type of cell that is reacting. For example, reactive B lymphocytes typically result in hyperplasia of the lymphoid follicles and germinal centers (follicular hyperplasia). Examples of diseases that are associated with follicular hyperplasia include chronic inflammation caused by organisms, rheumatoid arthritis, and AIDS. Lymph nodes from patients with AIDS have characteristic changes that initially show follicular hyperplasia with loss of mantle zones, intrafollicular hemorrhage ("follicle lysis"), and monocytoid B cell proliferation. Subsequently there will be depletion of lymphocytes (CD4+ lymphocytes) in both the follicles and the interfollicular areas. In contrast to reactive B cell processes, reactive T lymphocytes typically result in hyperplasia involving the T cell areas of the lymph node, namely the interfollicular regions and the paracortex. Examples of clinical situations associated with a T lymphocyte response include patients with viral infections, vaccinations, some drugs (particularly Dilantin), and systemic lupus erythematosus. Finally, the sinusoidal pattern of reaction involves expansion of the sinuses by benign macrophages as seen in reactive proliferations of the mononuclear-phagocytic system. Stellate microabscesses, irregular areas composed of central necrotic cellular and neutrophil debris surrounded by palisading macrophages, are characteristic of cat-scratch disease, lymphogranuloma venereum, and tularemia.

5-40. The answer is d. (*Cotran, 5/e, pp 213–214, 1285–1288.*) Duchenne muscular dystrophy (DMD) is a noninflammatory inherited myopathy that causes a progressive, severe weakness and degeneration of muscles, particularly the proximal muscles, such as the pelvic and shoulder girdles. The defective gene is located on the X chromosome and codes for dystrophin, a protein found on the inner surface on the sarcolemma. Histologically, the muscle fibers in patients with DMD show variations in

. size and shape, degenerative and regenerative changes in adjacent myocytes, necrotic fibers invaded by histiocytes, and progressive fibrosis. There are rounded, atrophic muscle fibers mixed with hypertrophied fibers. These muscle changes cause the creatine kinase levels in the serum to be elevated. The weak muscles are replaced by fibrofatty tissue, which results in pseudohypertrophy. In Duchenne's muscular dystrophy, symptoms begin before the age of 4, are progressive and lead to difficulty in walking, and are eventually followed by involvement of respiratory muscles, which causes death from respiratory failure before the age of 20. The classification of the muscular dystrophies is based on the mode of inheritance and clinical features. X-linked inheritance characterizes Duchenne's muscular dystrophy, autosomal dominant inheritance characterizes both myotonic dystrophy and fascioscapulohumeral type, while limb-girdle dystrophy is autosomal recessive. Sustained muscle contractions and rigidity (myotonia) are seen in myotonic dystrophy, the most common form of adult muscular dystrophy.

Dermatomyositis is an autoimmune disease that is one of a group of idiopathic inflammatory myopathies. The inflammatory myopathies are characterized by immune mediated inflammation and injury of skeletal muscle, and include polymyositis, dermatomyositis, and inclusion-body myositis. These diseases are associated with numerous types of autoantibodies, one of which is the anti-Jo-1 antibody. The capillaries are the principal target in patients with dermatomyositis. Damage is by complement-mediated cytotoxic antibodies against the microvasculature of skeletal muscle. In addition to proximal muscle weakness, patients typically develop a lilac discoloration around the eyelids with edema. Patients may also develop erythema over their knuckles (Gottron's sign). Histologically examination of muscles from patients with dermatomyositis reveal perivascular inflammation within the tissue around muscle fascicles This is in contrast to the other types of inflammatory myopathies, where the inflammation is within the muscle fascicles (endomysial inflammation). In particular, inclusion-body myositis is characterized by basophilic granular inclusions around vacuoles ("rimmed" vacuoles).

Werdnig-Hoffman disease is a severe lower motor neuron disease that presents in the neonatal period with severe proximal muscle weakness ("floppy infant").

5-41. The answer is a. (*Adams, 6/e, pp 676–678.*) The MRI of Susan's head revealed a pituitary microadenoma, a benign tumor arising from the anterior pituitary or adenohypophysis. This particular tumor consisted of cells that secrete the hormone prolactin, which is not only the stimulating factor for lactation but inhibits menstruation when levels are high. It is common for this tumor's symptoms to be manifested during the child-bearing years.

5-42. The answer is c. (*Kandel, 3/e, p 437. Adams, 6/e, pp 247–251.*) The visual problem is called bitemporal hemianopsia. Since the pituitary gland is in very close proximity to the optic chiasm, pituitary tumors often invade this structure. Since only the medial fibers (which perceive the temporal field of each eye) in each optic nerve cross, these are the fibers damaged by these tumors, and the patient will be unable to see either temporal visual field. Both central scotoma (an island of visual loss surrounded by normal vision in one eye), which is usually seen with lesions of the retina or optic nerve, and papilledema (blurring of the optic disc margin when viewed by funduscopic examination due to increased intracranial pressure) would not be caused by damage to the optic chiasm.

5-43. The answer is d. (*Kandel, 3/e, p 437.*) The optic chiasm can be compressed by pituitary tumors, causing bitemporal hemianopsia (see answer for previous question).

5-44. The answer is e. (*Kandel, 3/e, p 863.*) Prolactin-releasing factor is found in the arcuate nucleus of the hypothalamus, and activates the lactotrophic cells of the anterior pituitary gland.

5-45. The answer is c. (*Howard, 2/e, pp 680–681.*) Consumption of raw fish causes endemic diphyllobothriasis in Scandinavia and the Baltic countries. While most people do not become ill, a small percentage (2 percent) develop vitamin B12 deficiency anemia. The adult fish tapeworm has an affinity for vitamin B12 and may induce a serious megaloblastic anemia. Parvovirus B19 causes acute hemolytic anemia primarily in immunosuppressed patients. *Yersinia* infection is common in Scandinavia but is not fish-borne and does not cause anemia. The larval stage of *Taenia solium* is called cysticercus. Humans usually acquire cysticercosis by ingestion of food and water contaminated by infected human feces.

5-46. The answer is c. *(Fauci, 14/e, p 1984.)* This patient has a common presentation for secondary hypogonadism. The large tumor is inhibiting LH secretion, with consequently low testosterone secretion. No other pattern fits this clinical presentation.

5-47. The answer is d. *(Cotran, 5/e, pp 111–114, 679–680.)* An embolus is an intravascular solid, liquid, or gaseous mass that has been carried by the blood to a site away from where it was formed. Most emboli arise from thrombi and are called thromboemboli. These blood clots, most of which form in the deep veins of the lower extremities, may embolize to the lungs. The majority of small pulmonary emboli do no harm. If they are large enough, however, they may occlude the bifurcation of the pulmonary arteries and cause sudden death. This type of thromboembolus is called a saddle embolus. Arterial emboli most commonly originate within the heart from diseased valves (vegetations) or mural thrombi that are formed following myocardial infarctions. If there is a patent foramen ovale, a venous embolus may cross over through the heart to the arterial circulation producing an arterial (paradoxical) embolus.

There are several causes of non-thrombotic emboli. Fat emboli are associated with severe trauma and fractures of long bones. Fat emboli can be fatal because they can damage the endothelial cells and pneumocytes within the lungs, and produce adult respiratory distress syndrome (ARDS). Air emboli may be formed in decompression sickness, which is called Caisson's disease or the bends. Amniotic fluid emboli are associated with rupture of uterine venous sinuses and are a complication of childbirth. Amniotic fluid emboli may also lead to a fatal disease, disseminated intravascular coagulation (DIC), which is characterized by the combination of intravascular coagulation and hemorrhages. DIC results from the high thromboplastin activity of amniotic fluid.

5-48. The answer is b. *(Cotran, 5/e, pp 818–820, 823–825. Rubin, 2/e, pp 343, 696–697.)* Acute appendicitis, a disease found predominantly in adolescents and young adults, is characterized histologically by acute inflammatory cells, neutrophils, within the mucosa and muscular wall. Clinically, acute appendicitis causes right lower quadrant pain, nausea, vomiting, a mild fever, and a leukocytosis in the peripheral blood. These symptoms may not occur in the very young or the elderly. The inflamed appendiceal wall may become gangrenous and perforate in 24 to 48 h. Even with classic symptoms, the appendix may be histologically unremarkable in up to 20 percent of the cases. False positive diagnoses are to be preferred to the possible severe or fatal complications of a false negative diagnosis of acute appendicitis that results in rupture. Lymphoid hyperplasia with multinucleated giant cells (Warthin-Finkeldey giant cells) is characteristic of measles (rubeola). These changes can be found in the appendix, but this is quite rare. Dilatation of the lumen of the appendix is called a mucocele and may be caused by mucosal hyperplasia, a benign cystadenoma, or a malignant mucinous cystadenocarcinoma. If the latter tumor ruptures, it may seed the entire peritoneal cavity, causing the condition called pseudomyxoma peritonei. The most common tumor of the appendix is the carcinoid tumor. Grossly it is yellow in color and is typically located at the tip of the appendix. Histologically, carcinoids are composed of nests or islands of monotonous cells. Appendiceal carcinoids rarely metastasize.

5-49. The answer is d. (*Hardman and Limbird, 9/e, p 564. Katzung, 7/e, pp 363, 980.*) Flumazenil is a competitive antagonist of benzodiazepines at the γ-aminobutyric acid (GABA) receptor. Repeated administration is necessary because of its short half-life relative to that of most benzodiazepines.

5-50. The answer is e. (*Davis, 4/e, pp 705–706.*) Ornithosis (psittacosis) is caused by *Chlamydia psittaci.* Humans usually contract the disease from infected birds kept as pets or from infected poultry, including poultry in dressing plants. Although ornithosis may be asymptomatic in humans, severe pneumonia can develop. Fortunately, the disease is cured easily with tetracycline.

BLOCK 6

Answers

6-1. The answer e. *(Sierles, pp 76–79.)* Systematic desensitization can reduce anxiety in a situation by identify-ing a hierarchy of situations that produce anxiety from low to high. For example, the bridge designer can be taught progressive muscle relaxation until he is as relaxed as possible, at which point he will begin by driving across the shortest or least anxiety-producing bridge (in vivo exposure). As he successfully experiences crossing the lowest anxiety-producing bridge, he can proceed up the hierarchy of bridges until he masters crossing the most anxiety-producing bridge. This process of systematic desensitization can also be used cognitively if, after identifying the hierarchy, he can practice muscle relaxation, fantasize about crossing the lowest bridge without becoming anxious, and then proceed up the hierarchy. This principle can also be used to treat anxiety over such situations as going to the dentist or entering a crowded room, or a number of anxiety phobias. The muscle relaxation involves an important principle of reciprocal inhibition—a person cannot be relaxed and anxious simultaneously.

6-2. The answer is c. *(Fauci, 14/e, p 363.)* Any suspicious palpable mass should be biopsied despite a negative mammogram, which can happen from 10 to 15 percent of the time.

6-3. The answer is a. *(Kandel, 3/e, pp 831–832. Adams, 6/e, pp 456–457.)* Jane is not only unable to move her left side (hemiparesis), but ignores its existence (anosognosia or the syndrome of hemineglect). Even though she neglects her left side, the blink reflex should still be intact if she only neglects the side. Therefore, a visual field deficit called a homonymous hemianopsia is present on the left side, in which the left temporal and right nasal fields are damaged. There may also be some degree of primary sensory loss, which can be difficult to evaluate when a patient neglects the same side.

6-4. The answer is c. *(Adams, 6/e, pp 443–446, 456–457.)* Jane's deficits result from lesions of the posterior frontal cortex, as well as from some contribution of corticospinal tract fibers to the parietal lobe and deeper motor cortical structures. In addition, the neglect and hemisensory loss result from damage to the parietal cortex. The homonymous hemianopsia results from damage to the deep portion of the parietal lobe where the optic radiations pass to the superior and inferior banks of the visual cortex, causing the visual field defect.

6-5. The answer is d. (*Kandel, 3/e, p 1045.*) The posterior frontal lobe, as well as parietal lobe, are supplied by the middle cerebral artery. Areas supplied by this artery, such as primary and supplementary motor areas, and the primary and secondary somatosensory cortices may be effected. As a result, the patient may have left-sided weakness, upper motor neuron facial weakness that spares the forehead, and hemisensory loss.

6-6. The answer is e. (*Kandel, 3/e, p 1045.*) If the lesion is deep enough, the patient may have a visual field cut called a homonymous hemianopsia, where fibers traveling from the optic chiasm to the occipital cortex within the optic radiations are interrupted, and the patient doesn't see the left temporal and the right nasal visual field. It is common for patients with neglect not to notice the areas of blindness because they ignore the left side. Patients with this problem are usually advised not to drive a car.

6-7. The answer is d. (*Cotran, 5/e, pp 1023–1029.*) Benign enlargement of the prostate is caused by benign prostatic hyperplasia (BPH) and produces clinical symptoms of urinary frequency, nocturia, difficulty in starting and stopping urination, dribbling, and dysuria. Histologically the hyperplastic nodules are composed of a variable mixture of hyperplastic glands and hyperplastic stromal cells. Histologic signs of malignancy are not present. The development of BPH is associated with increased age and higher testosterone levels. BPH results from androgen-induced glandular proliferation, but estrogen also sensitizes the tissue to androgens. Urinary obstruction results as the inner, periurethral portions of the prostate (the middle and lateral lobes) are affected most commonly. BPH does not predispose the individual to cancer. In contrast to the benign histology of BPH, the histologic signs characteristic of prostatic adenocarcinoma include small glands that appear "back-to-back" without intervening stroma, or they appear to be infiltrating beyond the normal prostate lobules. Histologically these malignant glands are composed of a single layer of cuboidal epithelial cells, as the outer basal layer of epithelial cells, seen in normal and hyperplastic glands, is not present. These malignant cells often contain one or more enlarged nucleoli.

Inflammation of the prostate (prostatitis) is characterized by finding at least fifteen leukocytes per high power field in prostatic secretions. Prostatitis is classified as being either acute or chronic prostatitis. Patients with acute prostatitis present with fever, chills, and dysuria. It is usually caused by bacteria that cause urinary tract infections, such as *E. coli*. Chronic prostatitis presents clinically as low back pain, dysuria, and suprapubic discomfort. It is divided into chronic bacterial prostatitis, which is associated with recurrent urinary tract infections (UTI) with the same organism, and chronic abacterial prostatitis, which is not associated with recurrent UTIs. Instead chronic abacterial prostatitis is associated with infections with either *Chlamydia trachomatis* or *ureaplasma urealyticum*. Granulomatous prostatitis causes vague symptoms and has an unknown etiology. This diagnosis is made histologically.

6-8. The answer is d. *(Cotran, 5/e, pp 680–682.)* Many pathologic pulmonary changes can be found in the lungs of patients who expire under conditions of progressive, unexplained dyspnea, fatigue, and cyanosis. These changes range from pulmonary fibrosis to hypersensitivity pneumonitis and to recurrent, multiple pulmonary emboli. Furthermore, traditional hospital treatment modalities for progressive pulmonary deterioration (including high oxygen delivery, overhydration, lack of pulmonary ventilation, irregular ventilation by mechanical respiratory assistance [PEEP], and superimposed nosocomially acquired pneumonitis) can complicate pulmonary pathologic findings. However, unremitting, progressive dyspnea, cyanosis, and fatigue in a young female should suggest the diagnosis of primary pulmonary hypertension. Pulmonary vascular sclerosis is always associated with pulmonary hypertension primary or secondary to other states, such as emphysema and mitral stenosis.

6-9. The answer is e. *(Cotran, 5/e, p 309. Rubin, 2/e, pp 356–360, 384–385, 391–395, 1258.)* Numerous diseases result from bacterial infections of the oral cavity. *Actinomyces israelii*, a normal inhabitant of the mouth, is a branched, filamentous gram-positive bacteria that may produce an indurated (lumpy) jaw with multiple draining fistulas or abscesses. Small yellow colonies may be seen in the draining material, these being called sulfur granules. Scarlet fever, a disease of children, is caused by several strains of beta-hemolytic group A streptococci (*S. pyogenes*). An erythrogenic toxin damages vascular endothelium and produces a rash on the skin and oral mucosa. The tongue in a patient with scarlet fever may be fiery red with prominent papillae (raspberry tongue) or white-coated with hyperemic papillae (strawberry tongue). Acute necrotizing ulcerative gingivitis (Vincent angina or trench mouth) is caused by two symbiotic organisms, a fusiform bacillus and a spirochete (*Borrelia vincentii*), the combination being termed fusospirochetosis. *Corynebacterium diphtheriae* causes diphtheria, which is characterized by oral and pharyngeal pseudomembranes and a peripheral lymphocytosis. Rhinoscleroma, a chronic inflammation of the nose, is caused by *Klebsiella rhinoscleroma*, and histologically is characterized by numerous foamy macrophages, called Mikulicz cells.

6-10. The answer is d. (*Cotran, 5/e, pp 841–842. Chandrasoma, 3/e, pp 636–637.*) Despite various underlying causes, the clinical features of all types of liver failure are similar. A defective urea cycle results in hyperammonemia, while a foul-smelling breath (fetor hepaticus) is thought to occur due to volatile, sulfur-containing mercaptans being produced in the gut. If liver cell necrosis is present, serum hepatic enzymes, such as LDH, ALT, and AST, will be increased. Impaired estrogen metabolism in males can result in gynecomastia, testicular atrophy, palmar erythema, and spider angiomas of the skin. Additionally, deranged bilirubin metabolism results in jaundice (mainly conjugated hyperbilirubinemia) and a decreased synthesis of albumin (hypoalbuminemia) results in ascites. Symptoms of hepatic encephalopathy, a metabolic disorder of the neuromuscular system, include stupor, hyperreflexia, and asterixis, which describes a peculiar flapping tremor of the hands.

6-11. The answer is e. (*Cotran, 5/e, pp 67–70.*) Certain drugs are important in the control of acute inflammation because they inhibit portions of the metabolic pathways involving arachidonic acid. For example, corticosteroids induce the synthesis of lipocortins, a family of proteins that are inhibitors of phospholipase A_2. They decrease the formation of arachidonic acid and its metabolites, prostaglandins and leukotrienes. Aspirin, indomethacin, and other nonsteroidal anti-inflammatory drugs (NSAIDs), in contrast, inhibit cyclooxygenase and therefore inhibit the synthesis of prostaglandins and thromboxanes. The prostaglandins have several important functions. For example, prostaglandin E_2 (PGE_2), produced within the anterior hypothalamus in response to interleukin-1 secretion from leukocytes, results in fever. Therefore aspirin can be used to treat fever by inhibiting PGE_2 production. PGE_2 is also a vasodilator that can keep a ductus arteriosus open. At birth, breathing decreases pulmonary resistance and reverses the flow of blood through the ductus arteriosus. The oxygenated blood flowing from the aorta into the ductus inhibits prostaglandin production and closes the ductus arteriosus. Therefore prostaglandin E_2 can be given clinically to keep the ductus arteriosus open, while indomethacin can be used to close a patent ductus. Prostaglandin F_2 (PGF_2) causes uterine contractions, which can result in dysmenorrhea. Indomethacin can be used to treat dysmenorrhea by inhibiting the production of PGF_2.

Bradykinin is a nonapeptide that increases vascular· permeability, contracts smooth muscle, dilates blood vessels, and causes pain. It is part of the kinin system and is formed from high-molecular-weight kininogen (HMWK). Histamine, a vasoactive amine that is stored in mast cells, basophils, and platelets, acts on H_1 receptors to cause dilatation of arterioles and increased vascular permeability of venules.

6-12. The answer is c. (*DiPalma, 4/e, p 394. Hardman and Limbird, 9/e, pp 813–814.*) Digoxin is used in AF to slow the ventricular rate, not usually the AF itself. Digoxin acts to slow the speed of conduction, increase the atrial and AV nodal maximal diastolic resting membrane potential, and increase the effective refractory period in the AV node, which prevents transmission of all impulses from the atria to the ventricles. It exerts these effects by directly acting on the heart and by indirectly increasing vagal activity.

6-13. The answer is b. (*April, 3/e, pp 269–270.*) Inability of the thorax to expand and effectively lower intrathoracic (and hence, intrapleural) pressure on the affected side results in inadequate ventilation of the lung. Normal perfusion of an unventilated lung results in cyanosis owing to increased amounts of reduced hemoglobin in the arterial blood. Paralysis of either the right diaphragm or the right thoracic musculature alone would not normally produce cyanosis; at any rate, there is no indication that either of these factors is involved in the patient presented in the question.

6-14. The answer is d. (*Fauci, 14/e, pp 1993 and 2150.*) This patient has classic manifestations of hemochromatosis, which impairs hypothalamic pituitary function. Evaluation of serum ferritin is potentially diagnostic in this patient. All the other tests are not diagnostic for hemochromatosis.

6-15. The answer is a. (*Cotran, 5/e, pp 945–947. Rubin, 2/e, pp 828–831.*) In a young patient who presents with signs of edema, three renal diseases are in the differential diagnosis. These diseases have similar names and findings, which makes them easily confused with each other. For example, minimal change disease (MCD), focal segmental glomerulosclerosis (FSGS), and post-streptococcal glomerulonephritis may all produce the nephrotic syndrome, characterized by marked proteinuria. This finding can be documented by the presence of protein in a dipstick examination of the urine. MCD characteristically is associated with a selective proteinuria in which albumin is found in the urine rather than immunoglobulins. In contrast, FSGS is associated with a nonselective proteinuria. MCD is a selective proteinuria because it results from decreased amounts of polyanions (mainly heparan sulfate) in the glomerular basement membrane. These polyanions normally block the filtration of the small, but negatively charged albumin molecules. The glomeruli in patients with MCD lack electron dense deposits, and immunofluorescence (IF) tests are negative. These patients have no tendency to develop chronic renal failure, and they respond to steroid therapy. In contrast, FSGS has granular IgM and C3 deposits seen by IF, and patients do not respond to steroids. It is important to realize that FSGS, with no cellular proliferation, is different from focal segmental glomerulonephritis (FSGN), which has cellular proliferation, the main cause of FSGN being IgA (Berger's) nephropathy. Both MCD and FSGN have fusion of the foot processes of the podocytes that can be seen with electron microscopy, but since FSGS is focal and segmental, the biopsy specimen may not demonstrate other findings of FSGS that are not seen with MCD, such as thickening of the basement membrane with hyalinosis (the focal deposition of PAS positive material).

Although signs of the nephritic syndrome, such as hematuria, may be seen with FSGS, young children are more often found with acute post-streptococcal glomerulonephritis. This illness typically occurs 1 to 3 weeks after a group A, β-hemolytic streptococcal infection of the pharynx or skin, such as impetigo or scarlet fever. Patients develop hematuria, red cell casts, mild periorbital edema, and increased blood pressure. Laboratory tests reveal increased ASO titers and decreased C3. Cultures taken at the time of presentation with renal symptoms are negative. Light microscopy reveals diffuse endothelial and mesangial cell proliferation with neutrophil infiltration, so that narrowing of capillary lumens and enlargement of the glomerular tuft to fill Bowman's space occur. Electron microscopy reveals the mesangial deposits and large, hump-shaped subepithelial deposits in peripheral capillary loops that are characteristic. Immunofluorescence shows granular deposits containing IgG, C3, and often fibrin in glomerular capillary walls and mesangium. Children with post-streptococcal glomerulonephritis usually recover, and therapy is supportive only.

6-16. The answer is c. *(Rubin, 2/e, pp 310–313.)* Heavy metal poisoning may occur via the respiratory route owing to contaminated inhalant and vapors. Such poisoning is usually industrially related, as with mercury (calomel workers), arsenic (pesticides), and lead (batteries and paints). Cadmium has been implicated in producing not only an acute form of pneumonia, but, with chronic exposure to small concentrations of cadmium vapors, diffuse interstitial pulmonary fibrosis and an increased incidence of emphysema as well. The "honeycomb" radiologic pattern is indicative of an interstitial fibrotic process and may be the result of repeated pneumonitis and bronchitis. Cadmium can also be found in tobacco smoke. Cobalt poisoning leads to myocardiopathy, mercury poisoning leads to renal tubular damage, and lead poisoning leads to liver necrosis and cerebral edema. Arsenic poisoning, in addition to carrying an increased risk of lung and skin cancer, may cause death by inhibition of respiratory enzymes and cardiac subendocardial hemorrhages complicated by gastroenteritis with shock.

6-17. The answer is e. *(Cotran, 5/e, pp 994–995, 1007–1008. Damjanov, 10/e, pp 1710–1711, 2190–2191. Larsen, 1/e, pp 222–226.)* The cloaca is an embryonic structure that connects ventrally to the allantoic stalk and laterally to the mesonephric ducts. At about the eighth week of development a cloacal membrane forms within the cloaca and separates the cloaca into a dorsal rectum and a ventral urogenital sinus. The latter is the origin of the urachus, urinary bladder, and proximal urethra. Initially the urinary bladder is continuous with the allantois, which constricts and forms the thick, fibrous urachus. The urachus in turn becomes attenuated, but still remains attached to the bladder dome and forms the median umbilical ligament in the adult. Incomplete attenuation of the urachus (persistent urachus) can lead to formation of an urachal cyst, urachal sinus, or urachal fistula. The end attached to the bladder can remain and form a bladder diverticulum, while the central portion can remain and form an urachal cyst. Urachal sinuses and fistulas still connect the umbilicus to the urinary bladder, and therefore urine can leak at the site of the umbilicus.

Normally, mesodermal tissue grows onto the cloacal membrane to form the muscles of the lower abdominal wall. During this process the cloacal membrane is obliterated and disappears. In some embryos mesoderm does not grow onto the cloacal membrane. This leads to persistence of the cloacal membrane, which can become quite thin and rupture. This in turn causes the posterior bladder mucosa to evert through this defect in the anterior abdominal wall. This condition is called exstrophy and is associated with recurrent urinary infections and epispadias in males. There is also an increased incidence of neoplastic transformation, most commonly adenocarcinoma.

Meckel's diverticulum is a diverticulum found in the terminal ileum that is the result of persistence of the omphalomesenteric duct. It is usually about 2 inches long and is located less than 2 feet from the ileocecal valve. An omphalocele refers to protrusion of the intestines through an unclosed umbilical ring. This abnormality results from incomplete internalization of the intestines during fetal growth. A similar defect, gastroschisis, does not involve the umbilicus. Instead, viscera herniate through a defect in the anterior abdominal wall just lateral to the umbilicus.

Phimosis occurs when the orifice of the prepuce (foreskin) is too small to permit normal retraction. This may be due to inflammatory scarring or abnormal development of the prepuce. If a phimotic prepuce is forcibly retracted over the glans penis, a condition called paraphimosis may develop. This condition is extremely painful and may cause obstruction of the urinary tract or blood flow, which may lead to necrosis of the penis. Nonspecific infection of the glans and prepuce is called balanoposthitis. Genital malformations may cause an abnormal location of the urethral opening, either on the ventral surface of the penis (hypospadias) or the dorsal surface (epispadias). These abnormal developments may cause problems with infertility. Hypospadias is the result of failure of the urethral folds to close, while epispadias is the result of faulty positioning of the genital tubercle. The latter is also associated with exstrophy of the urinary bladder.

6-18. The answer is e. (*Cotran, 5/e, pp 1079–1084. Chandrasoma, 3/e, pp 811–814.*) Toxemia of pregnancy refers to the combination of hypertension, proteinuria, and pitting edema. This combination of signs is also called preeclampsia. When convulsions develop in an individual with preeclampsia the condition is then referred to as eclampsia. These signs and symptoms result from abnormal placental implantation with incomplete conversion of the blood vessels of the decidua. Both of these result in placental ischemia. Normally the blood vessels of the uterine wall at the site of implantation increase in diameter and lose their muscular components. These changes increase the blood flow to the placenta and are the result of increased production of prostacyclin (a strong vasodilator) and decreased production of thromboxane (a potent vasoconstrictor). These changes do not take place at the implantation site of patients who develop preeclampsia. This causes placental ischemia and damages the endothelial cells of the blood vessels of the placenta. This endothelial damage disrupts the normal balance between vasodilation and vasoconstriction. As a result, there are increased levels of vasoconstrictors, such as thromboxane, angiotensin, and endothelin, and decreased levels of vasodilators, such as PGI_2, PGE_2, and nitric oxide. This results in arterial vasoconstriction, which produces systemic hypertension, and can lead to activation of intravascular coagulation (DIC). Risk factors for the development of preeclampsia include nulliparity, twin gestation, and hydatidiform mole. Other complications associated with preeclampsia include renal disease and liver disease, such as the HELLP syndrome, which refers to hemolytic anemia, elevated liver enzymes, and low platelets.

6-19. The answer is a. (*Murray, 24/e, pp 216, 246–248, 266. Stryer, 4/e, pp 614–615, 687–689.*) Acetyl CoA carboxylase deficiency will drastically alter the ability of the patient to synthesize fatty acids. The fact that the infant was born at all is due to the body's ability to utilize fatty acids provided to it. However, all processes dependent upon *de novo* fatty acid biosynthesis will be affected. The lungs, in particular, require surfactant, a lipoprotein substance secreted by alveolar type II cells to function properly. Surfactant lowers alveolar surface tension facilitating gas exchange. It contains significant amounts of dipalmitoyl phosphatidylcholine. Palmitate is the major end product of *de novo* fatty acid synthesis. Acetyl CoA carboxylase formation of malonyl CoA is the first step of fatty acid synthesis. Biotin deficiency cannot be the problem since pyruvate carboxylase in gluconeogenesis is not affected. None of the other answers listed would have resulted in all of the symptoms given.

6-20. The answer is b. (*Hardman and Limbird, 9/e, pp 365–367.*) Benzodiazepines, such as diazepam, bind to the GABA receptor/ion channel complex, enhancing GABA-induced Cl⁻ currents related to more frequent bursts of Cl⁻ channel opening by GABA.

6-21. The answer is e. (*Cotran, 5/e, pp 163–164, 1289–1291. Damjanov, 10/e, pp 298–299.*) Almost all genes occur on chromosomes within the nucleus. There are a few genes, however, that are located within the mitochondria. These mitochondrial genes are found on mitochondrial DNA (mtDNA). These genes are all of maternal origin because ova have mitochondria within the large amount of cytoplasm, and sperm do not. This maternal origin means that mothers transmit all of the mtDNA to both male and female offspring, but only the daughters transmit it further. No transmission occurs through males. This mtDNA contains genes that mainly code for oxidative phosphorylation enzymes, such as NADH dehydrogenase, cytochrome c oxidase, and ATP synthase. Symptoms of deficiencies of these enzymes occur in organs that require large amounts of ATP, such as the brain, muscle, liver, and kidneys. The mtDNA of these patients may be composed of either a mixture of mutant and normal DNA (heteroplasmy) or of mutant DNA entirely (homoplasmy). The severity of these diseases correlates with the amount of mutant mtDNA that is present. One disease associated with mitochondrial inheritance is Leber hereditary optic neuropathy (LHON), characterized by progressive bilateral loss of central vision, which usually occurs between 15 and 35 years of age. Other examples of mitochondrial inheritance include mitochondrial myopathies, which are characterized by the presence of abnormal size and shaped mitochondria in muscle. These abnormal mitochondria may result in the histologic appearance of the muscle as being ragged red fibers. Electron microscopy reveals the presence within large mitochondria of rectangular crystals that have a "parking-lot" appearance.

6-22. The answer is b. (*Cotran, 5/e, p 641.*) T-cell lymphomas occurring in the thoracic cavity in young patients usually arise in the mediastinum and have a particularly aggressive clinical course with rapid growth in the mediastinum impinging upon the trachea or mainstem bronchi and leading to marked respiratory deficiency, which can in turn lead to death in a relatively short period of time if not treated. These unique lymphomas are characterized by rapid cell growth and spread into the circulation, where they produce elevated total white counts reflected by circulating lymphoma cells. As T cells they have characteristics of rosette formation with sheep blood cells. T cells also have subtypes and subsets, which can be delineated by monoclonal antibodies as CD4 helper, CD8 suppressor (cellular differentiation) T-cell surface antigens. The tumor cells also express IL-2 receptor. FC receptors occur on B cells and macrophages. Class II HLA antigens can be found on macrophages, Langerhans cells, and dendritic reticulum cells.

6-23. The answer is d. (*Cotran, 5/e, pp 1064–1065. Chandrasoma, 3/e, pp 764–767.*) Infertility affects close to 20 percent of married couples in the United States, and in many of these cases, the infertility is related to polycystic ovary (Stein-Leventhal) syndrome in the female. The symptoms of patients with this syndrome are related to increased androgen production, which causes hirsutism, and decreased ovarian follicle maturation, which can lead to amenorrhea. These patients typically have excess androgens (androstenedione), increased estrogen levels, increased LH levels, increased GnRH levels, and decreased FSH levels. The cause of this syndrome is thought to be the abnormal secretion of gonadotropins by the pituitary. Increased secretion of LH stimulates the thecal cells to secrete excess amounts of androgens, which are converted to estrone by the peripheral aromatization of androgens by the adrenal gland. Excess estrogens in turn increase the levels of gonadotropin-releasing hormone (GnRH), but decrease the levels of FSH. The GnRH increases the levels of LH, which then stimulate the theca cells of the ovary to secrete more androgens, and this hormonal cycle begins again. The ovaries in these patients are enlarged and have thick capsules, hyperplastic ovarian stroma, and numerous follicular cysts, which are lined by a hyperplastic theca interna. Since these patients do not ovulate there is a marked decreased number of corpora lutea, which in turn results in decreased progesterone levels. These patients also have an increased risk of developing endometrial hyperplasia and endometrial carcinoma because of the excess estrogen production. Treatment for these patients in the past involved surgical wedge resection of the ovary, but now treatment is with clomiphene, which stimulates ovulation.

6-24. The answer is b. (*Cotran, 5/e, pp 1055–1057.*) Dysfunctional uterine bleeding (DUB) is defined as abnormal uterine bleeding that is due to a functional abnormality rather than an organic lesion of the uterus. In contrast, secondary dysmenorrhea refers to painful menses associated with an organic cause, such as endometriosis, which is the most common cause. Most cases of DUB are related to an endocrine abnormality affecting the hypothalamic-pituitary-ovarian axis. The three main categories of DUB are anovulatory cycles (most common form), inadequate luteal phase, and irregular shedding. Anovulatory cycles consist of persistence of the graafian follicle without ovulation. This results in continued and excess estrogen production without the normal postovulatory rise in progesterone levels. With no progesterone production, no secretory endometrium is formed. Instead biopsies will reveal non-secretory (proliferative) endometrium with mild hyperplasia. The mucosa becomes too thick and is sloughed off, and this results in the abnormal bleeding. Anovulatory cycles characteristically occur at menarche and menopause. They are also associated with the poly-cystic ovary (Stein-Leventhal) syndrome. It is important to note that other causes of unopposed estrogen effect can lead to this appearance of a prolif-erative endometrium with mild hyperplasia. These causes include exoge-nous estrogen administration or estrogen-secreting neoplasms, such as a granulosa cell tumor of the ovary or an adrenal cortical neoplasm. If there is ovulation but the functioning of the corpus luteum is inadequate, then the levels of progesterone will be decreased. This will result in asynchrony between the chronologic dates and the histologic appearance of the secre-tory endometrium. This is referred to as an inadequate luteal phase (luteal phase defect) and is an important cause of infertility. Biopsies are usually performed several days after the predicted time of ovulation. If the his-tologic dating of the endometrium lags 4 of more days behind the chrono-logic date predicted by the menstrual history, the diagnosis of luteal phase defect can be made. Clinically these patients have low serum progesterone, FSH, and LH levels. In contrast to the above, prolonged functioning of the corpus luteum (persistent luteal phase with continued progesterone pro-duction) will result in prolonged heavy bleeding at the time of menses. Histologically there will be a combination of secretory glands mixed with proliferative glands (irregular shedding). Clinically these patients have regular periods, but the menstrual bleeding is excessive and prolonged (lasting 10 to 14 days). Current oral contraceptives, being a combination of estrogen and progesterone, will cause the endometrium to have inactive glands with predecidualized stroma. The endometrium from women who are postmenopausal will reveal an atrophic pattern with atrophic or inactive glands.

6-25. The answer is c. (*Cotran, 5/e, pp 219–231. Henry, 19/e, pp 708–709.*) Cytopenias occur in over 50 percent of patients with HIV infection either individually or as part of a pancytopenia. Suppression of hemopoiesis in the bone marrow as a result of mycobacterial, fungal, or protozoal infection; infiltration by lymphoma, leukemia, or Kaposi's sarcoma; and the effects of drugs (particularly zidovudine) may result in cytopenia. Anemia is seen in 80 to 85 percent of cases, usually in the pattern of anemia of chronic disease. Thrombocytopenia occurs in about 30 percent of cases and is thought to be a result of peripheral destruction of platelets, possibly by an immune mechanism. Neutropenia occurs in 40 percent of patients. Lymphopenia and a reduced ratio of CD4 to CD8 lymphocytes are characteristic of HIV infection. Atypical plasmacytoid lymphocytes are usually present in the peripheral blood smear. Examination of the bone marrow in cytopenic patients shows a normocellular or hypercellular pattern in more than 90 percent of cases.

6-26. The answer is a. (*Kandel, 3/e, p 785.*) June had a seizure, which began focally on the left motor strip (the left precentral gyrus), moved up the motor strip, then secondarily generalized, or spread, throughout the cortex. The phenomenon whereby there is twitching of an extremity that spreads to other areas on that extremity or other areas of the body is called a "Jacksonian march." This phenomenon is named for Hughlings Jackson, a neurosurgeon who was instrumental in mapping out the cerebral cortex and describing the somatotopic organization of the cortex of the prefrontal gyrus called a homunculus (meaning "little man"). Observing patients with a Jacksonian march helped him to identify areas represented at each location of the motor strip.

6-27. The answer is c. (*Kandel, 3/e, p 789.*) Very often, there is inhibition following a seizure, which accounts for drowsiness or a "post-ictal state" after the seizure has finished. Sometimes, epileptic discharges spread to other areas of the cortex, recruiting contiguous areas of cortex through callosal, commissural, and sometimes thalamic circuits to eventually involve a large area of the cortex, causing the movements of the entire body. This occurs with a generalized seizure. If the cortex of both hemispheres become involved, there may be impairment or loss of consciousness. The cells (often pyramidal cells) in the cortex can generate a seizure through high-frequency, synchronous discharges in large groups. If the seizure begins focally, as this one did, there may be a "Todd's paralysis," as June had, where there is transient paralysis of the involved motor area during the post-ictal period.

6-28. The answer is e. *(Kandel, 3/e, p 785.)* There is somatotopic organization of the motor strip (see answer for Question 6-27), and cortical neurons are included among the most likely to generate seizures, making this area the most likely to cause such a pattern.

6-29. The answer is e. *(Kandel, 3/e, pp 782–787.)* The pyramidal cell is a cell in the cortex that uses glutamate, an excitatory neurotransmitter, whereas most other types of cortical neurons use GABA, an inhibitory neurotransmitter. The spike, one identifying feature of an epileptic seizure seen on electroencephalogram recorded on the scalp, is initiated by a depolarization shift, which is thought to be generated by excitatory post-synaptic potentials.

6-30. The answer is a. *(Levinson, Jawetz, 4/e, pp 128–129.)* Mycoplasma pneumoniae causes a respiratory infection known as "primary atypical pneumonia" or "walking pneumonia." Although disease caused by *M. pneumoniae* can be contracted year round, thousands of cases occur during the winter months in all age groups. The disease, if untreated, will persist for 2 weeks or longer. Rare but serious side effects include cardiomyopathies and central nervous system complications. Infection with *M. pneumoniae* may be treated with either erythromycin or tetracycline. The organism lacks a cell wall and so is resistant to the penicillin and the cephalosporin groups of antibiotics.

6-31. The answer is e. *(Fauci, 14/e, p 1975.)* Men frequently present with marked hyperprolactinemia from a macroadenoma. Presenting manifestations typically are sexual dysfunction and decreased libido. The prolactin causes a decrease in LH and a concomitant decrease in testosterone. Thus, the patient will have a high prolactin level associated with low LH and low testosterone levels. The pattern of low testosterone, high LH, and low prolactin is typical of primary hypergonadism.

6-32. The answer is d. *(Cotran, 5/e, pp 616–623. Henry, 19/e, pp 725–726, 729–736, 740–743.)* Abnormalities of blood vessels (capillary fragility) or platelets can be detected by either the tourniquet test or the bleeding time. These tests do not test the coagulation cascade. In contrast, the platelet count and platelet morphology are both useful in evaluating platelet abnormalities, while the prothrombin time (PT) and the partial thromboplastin time (PTT) measure the coagulation cascade. The PT measures the extrinsic pathway, while the PTT measures the intrinsic coagulation pathway.

An abnormal tourniquet test and bleeding time with a normal PTT and PT may be caused by either blood vessel abnormalities or platelet abnormalities. Blood vessel abnormalities and abnormal platelet function have normal platelet counts (choice "A" in table). Causes of blood vessel abnormalities include decreased vitamin C (scurvy) and vasculitis, while causes of platelet dysfunction include the Bernard-Soulier syndrome and Glanzmann's thrombasthenia. A decrease in the platelet count (choice "C" in the table) indicates thrombocytopenia and can be seen in patients with ITP. Normal platelet counts with normal bleeding times are suggestive of abnormalities of the coagulation cascade. A prolonged PTT only (choice "B" in the table) is seen with abnormalities of the intrinsic pathway, such as hemophilia A or B. A prolonged PT only (choice "D" in the table) is seen with abnormalities of the extrinsic pathway, such as a deficiency of factor VII. A prolongation of both PTT and PT is seen with liver disease, vitamin K deficiency, and DIC. Deficiencies of the vitamin K-dependent factors, such as induced with Coumadin therapy or broad-spectrum antibiotic therapy, are associated with a normal tourniquet test, bleeding time, and platelet count, but there will be a markedly increased PT, and the PTT may be increased or normal (also choice "D" in the table). Therefore, the PT is used as a screening test to monitor patients taking oral Coumadin. A prolonged bleeding time with a normal platelet count, but a prolonged PTT (choice "E" in table) is highly suggestive of von Willebrand disease.

6-33. The answer is d. (*Gelehrter, pp 129–131. Isselbacher, 13/e, pp 348–349. Jorde, pp 210–215. Scriver, 7/e, pp 367–399. Thompson, 5/e, pp 298–301.*) Glucose-6-phosphate dehydrogenase (G6PD) deficiency is probably the most common genetic disease, affecting more than 400 million people worldwide. Tropical African and Mediterranean peoples exhibit the highest prevalence because the disease, like sickle cell trait, confers resistance to malaria. More than 400 types of abnormal G6PD alleles have been described, meaning that most affected individuals will be compound heterozygotes. The phenotype of jaundice and red blood cell hemolysis with anemia is triggered by a variety of infections and drugs, including a dietary substance in fava beans.

Sulfanilamide and related antibiotics as well as antimalarial drugs are notorious for inducing hemolysis in G6PD-deficient individuals. G6PD deficiency exhibits X-linked recessive inheritance, explaining why three males but not the parents would become ill when exposed to antimalarials.

6-34. The answer is b. (*DiPalma, 4/e, p 738. Hardman and Limbird, 9/e, p 1062.*) Sulfonamides should not be used in pregnant women at term because of their ability to cross the placenta and enter the fetus in concentrations sufficient to produce toxic effects. Sulfonamides should also not be given to neonates, especially premature infants, because they compete with bilirubin for serum albumin binding, resulting in increased levels of free bilirubin, which causes kernicterus.

6-35. The answer is a. (*Cotran, 5/e, pp 162–163.*) Fragile X syndrome is one of four diseases that are characterized by long repeating sequences of three nucleotides. The other diseases are Huntington disease, myotonic dystrophy, and spinal and bulbar muscular atrophy. The fragile X syndrome, which is more common in males than females, is one of the most common causes of familial mental retardation. Additional clinical features of this disorder include developmental delay, a long face with a large mandible, large everted ears, and large testicles (macro-orchidism). Examination of the DNA from patients with fragile X syndrome reveals multiple tandem repeats of the nucleotide sequence CGG on the X chromosome. Normally these repeats average up to 50 in number, but in patients with fragile X syndrome there are more than 230 repeats. This number of repeats is called a full mutation. Normal transmitting males (NTM) and carrier females have between 50 to 230 CGG repeats. This number of repeats is called a premutation. During oogenesis, but not spermatogenesis, premutations can be converted to mutations by amplification of the triplet repeats. This explains the much higher incidence of mental retardation in grandsons rather than brothers of normal transmitting males (Sherman's paradox), as the premutation is amplified in females, but not in males. Since the premutation is not amplified in males, no daughters of NTM are affected. An additional finding associated with these repeat units is anticipation, which refers to the fact that the disease is worse with subsequent generations.

6-36. The answer is b. (*McPhee, 2/e, p 551; Fauci, 14/e, pp 1446 and 2092.*) Kartagener's syndrome is also known as the immotile cilia syndrome.

Asthenospermia—poor sperm motility—is due to missing dynein arms, the basic defect of Kartagener's syndrome. Kartagener's syndrome has no effect on sperm count or the basic anatomy of the male reproductive tract.

6-37. The answer is b. (*Wilson-Pauwels, pp 26–33.*) The third cranial nerve (oculomotor) controls four of the six extraocular muscles that move the eye. When this nerve fails to function, the eye remains deviated laterally due to the unopposed action of the other two extraocular muscles. When the eyes no longer move together, patients have double vision because the visual cortex now receives two different images. In addition, fibers originating in the third nerve nucleus innervate the levator palpebrae superioris, a muscle which helps to lift the eyelid. Damage to the optic nerve causes loss of vision, blurred vision, and a central scotoma (blind spot in the center of the visual field). Damage to the cervical sympathetic fibers causes *Horner's syndrome*, consisting of ptosis (drooping of the eyelid), miosis (constriction of the pupil), and anhydrosis (loss of sweating), not eye movement abnormalities. The actions of the superior oblique, (the muscle innervated by the trochlear nerve) include intorsion, depression, and abduction. The abducens nerve mediates the lateral rectus muscle, which abducts the eye.

6-38. The answer is c. (*Wilson-Pauwels, pp 26–33.*) The eye is depressed and abducted due to the unopposed actions of the superior oblique and lateral rectus muscles, which together move the eye downward, and abduct it (see Answer 6-37 for the actions of these muscles). The other four muscles are innervated by the oculomotor nerve, which presumably has been damaged.

6-39. The answer is e. (*Kandel, 3/e, p 728. Adams, 6/e, p 795.*) This is an example of Weber syndrome, or a lesion involving the third cranial nerve outflow tract, and the corticospinal and corticobulbar tracts in the cerebral peduncles of the midbrain. Weber syndrome may occur as a result of an occlusion of the interpeduncular branches of the posterior cerebral artery which supply this portion of the midbrain, a tumor pressing on this area, an aneurysm (circumscribed dilation of an artery) of the posterior communicating artery, or a plaque (lesion) related to multiple sclerosis.

6-40. The answer is c. (*Wilson-Pauwels, pp 34–36.*) Fibers from the Edinger-Westphal nucleus are affected by a lesion of the midbrain, as well, and because they are instrumental in constricting the pupil, this lesion causes the patient to have a dilated pupil. If there is a mass external to the midbrain, but pressing on the oculomotor nerve, then the preganglionic parasympathetic fibers traveling to the ciliary ganglion—which in turn, innervate the pupillary constrictor muscles—can be damaged, also causing a dilated pupil. Cervical sympathetic fibers cause pupillary dilatation, so damage to these fibers causes pupillary constriction (see Horner's syndrome, above).

6-41. The answer is b. *(Hardman and Limbird, 9/e, p 444.)* This patient ate tyramine-rich foods while taking an MAOI and went into hypertensive crisis. Tyramine causes release of stored catecholamines from presynaptic terminals, which can cause hypertension, headache, tachycardia, cardiac arrhythmias, nausea, and stroke. In patients who do not take MAOIs, tyramine is inactivated in the gut by MAO, and patients taking MAOIs must be warned about the dangers of eating tyramine-rich foods.

6-42. The answer is d. *(Fauci, 14/e, pp 628–629.)* Any back pain in a patient with a known history of carcinoma should be evaluated for the possibility of spinal cord disease.

6-43. The answer is d. *(Baum, 3/e, pp 219–220.)* Uncontrollable bouts of pain are most apt to be the patient's major source of stress. She probably feels that she could cope with her slowly developing disability and loss of self-esteem if she could have relief from or control over the bouts of pain. She may know that about 60 percent of patients with rheumatoid arthritis become progressively disabled and that there is no cure for the disease. Pain is more severe among patients who are anxious or depressed. She must somehow learn how to cope with the pain, swelling, and fatigue.

Staying busy tends to be an effective way of distracting attention from the pain. Concern for her future could also be very much on her mind as she sees and feels the chronic, progressive, and debilitating aspect of her disease and becomes increasingly concerned for her future welfare, care, and loss of independence. Some behavioral and cognitive behavioral approaches could be effective in reducing the patient's pain and distress, along with stress management and coping skill instruction.

6-44. The answer is b. *(Cotran, 5/e, pp 550–554. Chandrasoma, 3/e, pp 349–353.)* Infective endocarditis is the result of micro-organisms growing on any of the heart valves. These organisms may have either high virulence or low virulence. Highly virulent organisms, such as *Staphylococcus aureus* and group A streptococci, infect previously normal valves and produce severe symptoms within six weeks. This abnormality is referred to as acute bacterial endocarditis. In contrast, organisms of low virulence, such as α-hemolytic viridans streptococci and *Staphylococcus epidermis*, infect previously damaged valves, such as valves damaged by rheumatic fever. These organisms produce symptoms that last longer than six weeks. This abnormality is referred to as subacute bacterial endocarditis. Infective endocarditis in IV drug abusers, which normally occurs on the tricuspid valve, is caused by *Staphylococcus aureus*, group A streptococci, *Candida* species, and gram-negative bacilli like *Pseudomonas* species. Symptoms in patients with infective endocarditis are the result of bacteremia, emboli from the vegetations, immune complexes, and valvular disease. Bacteremia produces fever, positive blood cultures (several of which may be needed for confirmation), abscesses, and osteomyelitis. Embolization of parts of the large, friable vegetations can produce Roth spots in the retina, splinter hemorrhages in nail beds, and infarcts of the brain, heart, and spleen. Splenic infarcts will produce left upper quadrant (LUQ) abdominal pain. Immune complexes can deposit in multiple areas of the body and cause glomerulonephritis, vasculitis, tender nodules in the fingers and toes (Osler's nodes), and red papules in the palms and soles (Janeway lesions). Valvular disease can also result in perforation and valvular regurgitation.

6-45. The answer is c. (*Cotran, 5/e, pp 451–454.*) Cystic fibrosis (CF) is one of the most common lethal genetic diseases that affects white populations (1/2000). The primary abnormality in patients with cystic fibrosis involves the epithelial transport of chloride. Normally, binding of a ligand to a membrane surface receptor activates adenyl cyclase, which leads to increased intracellular cAMP. This in turn activates protein kinase A, which phosphorylates the cystic fibrosis transmembrane conductance regulator (CFTR), causing it to open and release chloride ions. Sodium ions and water then follow the chloride ions to maintain the normal viscosity of mucus. The most common abnormality in patients with CF involves decreased glycosylation of the CFTR, which then does not become incorporated into the cell membrane. A lack of chloride channels then causes decreased chloride, sodium, and water secretion, all of which together results in a very thick mucus (the other name of CF is "mucoviscidosis"). These thick mucus plugs can block the pancreatic ducts, which causes fibrosis and cystic dilatation of the ducts (hence the name "cystic fibrosis"). Decreased excretion of pancreatic lipase leads to malabsorption of fat and steatorrhea, which may lead to deficiency of fat soluble vitamins. Thick mucus may also cause intestinal obstruction in neonates, a condition called meconium ileus. Abnormal mucus in the pulmonary tree leads to atelectasis, fibrosis, bronchiectasis, and recurrent pulmonary infections, especially with *S. aureus* and *Pseudomonas* species. Obstruction of the vas deferens and seminal vesicles in males leads to sterility, while obstruction of the bile duct will produce jaundice. This child's skin tasted salty because of increased sweat electrolytes, the result of decreased reabsorption of electrolytes from the lumens of sweat ducts.

6-46. The answer is a. (*Cotran, 5/e, pp 213–214, 1289–1291, 1292. Rubin, 2/e, pp 1359–1361, 1364–1365, 1370.*) Myasthenia gravis is an acquired autoimmune disease with circulating antibodies to the acetylcholine receptors at the myoneural junction. These antibodies cause abnormal muscle fatigability, which typically involves the extraocular muscles and leads to ptosis and diplopia. Other muscles may also be involved, and this may cause many different symptoms, such as problems with swallowing. Two-thirds of patients with myasthenia gravis have thymic abnormalities; the most common is thymic hyperplasia. A minority of patients have a thymoma. Lack of lactate production during ischemic exercise is seen in metabolic diseases of muscle caused by a deficiency of myophosphorylase. Dermatomyositis is an autoimmune disease produced by complement-mediated cytotoxic antibodies against the microvasculature of skeletal muscle. Rhabdomyolysis is destruction of skeletal muscle that releases myoglobin into the blood. This may cause myoglobinuria and acute renal failure. Rhabdomyolysis may follow an influenza infection, heat stroke, or malignant hyperthermia. Corticosteroid therapy may cause muscle weakness and selective type 2 atrophy.

6-47. The answer is b. (*Jawetz, 19/e, pp 314–316.*) Hairs infected with *Microsporum canis* and *M. audouini* both fluoresce with a yellow-green color under Wood's light, while *Trichophyton rubrum*, *T. tonsurans*, and *Epidermophyton floccosum* do not. But *M. audouini* is an anthropophilic agent of tinea capitis, whereas *M. canis* is zoophilic. *M. canis* is primarily seen in children and is associated with infected cats or dogs.

6-48. The answer is a. *(Fauci, 14/e, p 1984.)* This patient most typically has Kallmann's syndrome, which is a deficiency in the secretion of LHRH from the hypothalamus. Typically, these patients will respond to LHRH, although they may need LHRH priming. Testosterone will be low from the lack of LHRH stimulation of LH secretion.

6-49. The answer is d. *(Cotran, 5/e, pp 324–327, 694–698, 700–703.)* Tuberculosis (TB) is caused by infection with *Mycobacterium tuberculosis*. Mycobacteriaceae are slow growing aerobic rods, with cell walls rich in glycolipids, true waxes, and long chain fatty acids called mycolic acids. The lipid rich mycolic acid containing cell wall is responsible for the unique staining properties of the *Mycobacteria*, namely their impermeability to most basic dyes and their resistance to acid decolorization (acid-fast staining). Infection with *M. tuberculosis* occurs either as a primary infection or a secondary reactivation or reinfection. The initial infection of primary tuberculosis, the Ghon complex, consists of a subpleural lesion near the fissure between the upper and lower lobes and enlarged caseous lymph nodes that drain the pulmonary lesion. The histologic lesions of TB reveal caseating granulomas with Langerhans giant cells. Although primary pulmonary tuberculosis is usually asymptomatic, systemic and localizing symptoms can occur. These symptoms include malaise, anorexia, weight loss, fever, night sweats, cough, and hemoptysis. The pulmonary lesion of secondary tuberculosis is usually located in the apex of one of both lungs. Progressive pulmonary tuberculosis may result in cavitary fibrocaseous tuberculosis, miliary tuberculosis, or tuberculous bronchopneumonia. Miliary tuberculosis consists of multiple small yellow-white lesions scattered throughout the entire lung. These lesions are the result of erosion of a granulomatous lesion into a blood vessel with subsequent lymphohematogenous dissemination. While TB is often asymptomatic, the resultant hypersensitivity reaction is a marker for infection in those individuals without clinically apparent disease. The TB skin test is called the Mantoux Test and is characterized by the intradermal injection of PPD (purified protein derivative). An area of ½ cm or more in diameter of induration at 48 hours is a positive result. The diagnosis of TB depends upon the clinical picture and chest x-ray. Acid-fast stains of sputum are followed with culture, not only to identify the species of mycobacteria but to determine the pattern of antibiotic sensitivity. Treatment is with isoniazid (INH) combined with other antibiotics.

Klebsiella pneumoniae is a cause of bacterial pneumonia in debilitated and malnourished individuals, such as chronic alcoholics. Patients develop a thick, gelatinous sputum production. This bacterial infection has a greater mortality than pneumococcal pneumonia. Legionnaires' disease is a form of bronchopneumonia that is caused by the gram-negative bacillus, *Legionella pneumophila*. This organism is almost ubiquitous in water and is spread by inhalation of contaminated airborne droplets. Infection results in a patchy bronchopneumonia, and microscopically the alveolar spaces are filled with an inflammatory exudate of neutrophils and macrophages. There may be multiple, small areas of necrosis and abscess. Organisms cannot be visualized by routine stains, so instead a Dieterle silver stain is used.

6-50. The answer is c. (*McPhee, 2/e, pp 544–548; Fauci, 14/e, pp 2088 and 2091–2092.*) Androgen insensitivity can present as an inability for a male child to go into puberty. Low FSH and LH levels are expected to yield low testosterone levels. High FSH and LH levels are usually markers of end-organ damage and lack of feedback of testosterone on the pituitary due to low testosterone levels. Puberty can be delayed by hyperthyroidism, with FSH and LH levels usually appropriate to the testosterone level. An XXY karyotype (Klinefelter's) often has no effect on testosterone level.

BLOCK 7

Answers

7-1. The answer is b. *(Gelehrter, pp 57–65. Isselbacher, 13/e, pp 347–349. Jorde, pp 185–209. Scriver, 7/e, pp 79–80. Thompson, 5/e, pp 349–363.)* A pattern of major or minor anomalies is known as a syndrome. The child's minor abnormalities plus developmental delay are strongly suggestive of a syndrome. It is important to distinguish syndromes from sequences (i.e., multiple consequences produced by a single embryologic error) or isolated birth defects (i.e., disruptions, deformations, and malformations) since the latter categories usually have an optimistic prognosis with minimum recurrence risk.

7-2. The answer is d. *(DiPalma, 4/e, pp 489–490. Hardman and Limbird, 9/e, pp 668–669.)* Cromolyn inhibits the release of mediators from mast cells, including histamine and slow-reacting substance of anaphylaxis (SRS-A), which prevents allergically induced bronchospasm. Cromolyn is of no use in an acute asthmatic attack, but is of considerable help in asthma prophylaxis, particularly in children.

7-3. The answer is b. *(Cotran, 5/e, pp 1219–1227. Chandrasoma, 3/e, pp 963–966.)* Osteopenia (reduction in the amount of bone) is seen in osteoporosis, osteomalacia, and osteitis fibrosa. Osteoporosis is characterized by qualitatively normal bone that is decreased in amount. Histologic bone sections reveal thin trabeculae that have normal calcification and normal osteoblasts and osteoclasts. Osteoporosis predisposes patients to fractures of weight-bearing bones, such as the femur and vertebral bodies. Patients typically have normal serum levels of calcium, phosphorus, alkaline phosphatase, and parathyroid hormone. Osteoporosis is classified as being primary or secondary. Primary osteoporosis, the most common type of osteoporosis, occurs most often in postmenopausal women and has been related to decreased estrogen levels. Cigarette smoking is also associated with an increased incidence of osteoporosis. Clinically significant osteoporosis is related to the maximum amount of bone a person has (peak bone mass), which is largely genetically determined. Secondary osteoporosis develops secondary to many conditions such as corticosteroid administration, hyperthyroidism, and hypogonadism.

Osteopetrosis is a rare inherited disease having abnormal, decreased functioning osteoclasts. This abnormality results in reduced bone resorption and abnormally thickened bone. In these patients, multiple fractures are frequent as the bones are structurally weak and abnormally brittle. Increased fragility of bones is also present in osteomalacia (caused by abnormal vitamin D metabolism in adults), and osteitis deformans (Paget's disease). Osteitis fibrosa cystica (von Recklinghausan's disease of bone) is seen with severe hyperparathyroidism and is characterized by increased bone cell activity, peritrabecular fibrosis, and cystic bone lesions.

7-4. The answer is c. (*Cotran, 5/e, pp 85–87.*) Tissue repair occurs through the regeneration of damaged cells and the replacement of tissue by connective tissue. Tissue repair involves the formation of granulation tissue, which histologically is characterized by a combination of proliferating fibroblasts and proliferating blood vessels. Proliferating cells are cells that are rapidly dividing and usually have prominent nucleoli. This histologic feature should not be taken as a sign of dysplasia or malignancy. It is important not to confuse the term granulation tissue with the similar sounding term granuloma. The latter term refers to a special type of inflammation that is characterized by the presence of activated macrophages (epithelioid cells). One aspect of tissue repair involves wound healing, which occurs by either primary union or secondary union. Primary intention refers to healing of a clean sutured surgical incision. Healing by secondary intention differs from healing by primary intention in that it involves more initial tissue damage, more inflammatory response, takes longer to clear away debris, takes longer to granulate in, and contraction of the scar is a major factor in healing.

7-5. The answer is e. (*Cotran, 5/e, pp 443–444. Rubin, 2/e, pp 209–211.*) TORCH is an acronym referring to a group of microorganisms that produce similar changes during fetal or neonatal infection. The T stands for toxoplasma, the O for others, the R for rubella, the C for cytomegalovirus, and the H for herpes simplex virus. The "others" include syphilis, tuberculosis, and many other microorganisms. Manifestations of the TORCH complex include brain lesions, such as encephalitis and intracranial calcifications; ocular defects, including chorioretinitis; and cardiac abnormalities. Children born with congenital syphilis, caused by maternal infection with *Treponema pallidum*, initially show changes typical of the TORCH complex, but later they may develop characteristic lesions including flattening of the nose (saddle nose), notched incisors (Hutchinson's teeth), malformed molars (mulberry molars), outward bowing of the anterior tibia (saber shins), and progressive vascularization of the cornea (interstitial keratitis). The combination of deafness, interstitial keratitis, and notched incisors is referred to as Hutchinson's triad.

7-6. The answer is d. *(Adams, 6/e, p 347.)* The CT scan of Louise's brain revealed a large, acute stroke of her upper pons and midbrain. Strokes of these areas often result from occlusion of the basilar artery and can produce coma, or a variant of hypersomnia called akinetic mutism or coma vigil. An EEG of a patient like this shows a pattern associated with slow wave sleep, but eye movements are preserved.

7-7. The answer is a. *(Kandel, 3/e, p 1047.)* It is likely that the corticospinal tracts within the pons were damaged during this very large stroke, causing the increased tone from lack of inhibition, as well as the lack of movement in Louise's arms and legs.

7-8. The answer is d. *(Kandel, 3/e, pp 726–728, 815–816.)* Infarctions of perforators of the basilar artery, supplying the reticular formation of the pons, may cause coma. These perforators also supply the corticospinal tracts, causing the increased tone and weakness of Louise's legs, so a large stroke may involve both functions.

7-9. The answer is c. *(Adams, 6/e, p 350.)* Coma occurs because there is damage to the brainstem tegmentum, which is a major component of the ascending reticular activating system. Although it is not known exactly which area is precisely responsible for consciousness, lesions of this region, as well as projections from the medial regions of the midbrain reticular formation, can produce coma.

7-10. The answer is d. *(Fauci, 14/e, p 620.)* Ectopic acromegaly is a paraneoplastic disorder related to cancer, including that of the lung. Conversely, hypercalcemia, hypercortisolism, and hypophosphatemia also are disorders associated with lung cancer.

7-11. The answer is c. (*McPhee, 2/e, pp 530 and 539; Fauci 14/e, pp 812–817.*) Pelvic inflammatory disease is a cause of tubal scarring, setting the stage for an ectopic (tubal) pregnancy. As the pregnancy grows, the tube is stretched, causing pain. Endometriosis causes pain with each menstrual cycle, which is not the case here. Urinary tract infection can cause pain, but she would be expected to have dysuria. Placental abruption occurs only after 20 weeks of pregnancy. She is clearly not premenstrual, because she is pregnant.

7-12. The answer is d. (*Cotran, 5/e, pp 849–856. Chandrasoma, 3/e, pp 643–645.*) Several clinical syndromes may develop after exposure to any of the viruses that cause hepatitis, including asymptomatic hepatitis, acute hepatitis, fulminant hepatitis, chronic hepatitis, and the carrier state. Asymptomatic infection in individuals is documented by serologic abnormalities only. Liver biopsies in patients with acute hepatitis, either the anicteric phase or the icteric phase, will reveal focal necrosis of hepatocytes (forming Councilman bodies) and lobular disarray resulting from ballooning degeneration of the hepatocytes. These changes are nonspecific, but the additional finding of fatty change is suggestive of hepatitis C virus (HCV) infection. Clinically acute viral hepatitis is classified into three phases. During the prodrome phase, patients may develop symptoms that include anorexia, nausea and vomiting, headaches, photophobia, and myalgia. An unusual symptom associated with acute viral hepatitis is altered olfaction and taste, especially the loss of taste for coffee and cigarettes. The next phase, the icteric phase, involves increased bilirubin-producing jaundice. Patients may also develop light stools and dark urine (due to disrupted bile flow), and ecchymoses (due to decreased vitamin K). The final phase is the convalescence phase. Fulminant hepatitis refers to massive necrosis and is seen in about 1 percent of patients with either hepatitis B or C, but very rarely with hepatitis A infection. The biggest risk for fulminant hepatitis is coinfection with both hepatitis B and D. Finally, chronic hepatitis is defined as elevated serum liver enzymes for longer than 6 months. Patients may be either symptomatic or asymptomatic.

7-13. The answer is c. (*Cotran, 5/e, pp 861–866. Chandrasoma, 3/e, pp 655–658.*) Abnormalities of metabolism are associated with a diverse group of liver disease. Hemochromatosis, excessive accumulation of body iron, may be primary or secondary. Primary hemochromatosis is a genetic disorder of iron metabolism that is inherited as an autosomal recessive disorder. The classic clinical triad for this disease consists of micronodular pigment cirrhosis, diabetes mellitus, and skin pigmentation. The combination of diabetes and skin pigmentation is called "bronze diabetes." In the majority of patients the serum iron is above 250 mg/dL, serum ferritin is above 500 ng/dL, and iron (transferrin) saturation approaches 100 percent. In patients with primary hemochromatosis, the excess iron is deposited in the cytoplasm of parenchymal cells of many organs, including the liver and pancreas. Liver deposition of iron leads to cirrhosis, which in turn increases the risk of hepatocellular carcinoma. Iron deposition in the islets of the pancreas leads to diabetes mellitus. Iron deposition in the heart leads to congestive heart failure, which is the major cause of death in these patients. Iron deposition in the joints leads to arthritis, while deposition in the testes leads to atrophy. Secondary hemochromatosis, also called systemic hemosiderosis, is most common in patients with hemolytic anemias, such as thalassemia. Excess iron may also be due to an excess number of transfusions, or increased absorption of dietary iron. In idiopathic (primary) hemochromatosis iron accumulates in the cytoplasm of parenchymal cells, but in secondary hemochromatosis the iron is deposited in the mononuclear phagocytic system. In both conditions the iron is deposited as hemosiderin, which stains an intense blue color with the Prussian blue stain. Since the iron deposition does not usually occur in the parenchymal cells in secondary hemochromatosis, there usually is no organ dysfunction or injury.

Reyes syndrome (RS) is an acute postviral illness that is seen mainly in children. It is characterized by encephalopathy, microvesicular fatty change of the liver, and widespread mitochondrial injury. Electron microscopy (EM) reveals large budding or branching mitochondria. The mitochondrial injury results in decreased activity of the citric acid cycle and urea cycle and defective beta-oxidation of fats, which then leads to the accumulation of serum fatty acids. The typical patient presents several days after a viral illness with pernicious vomiting. RS is associated with hyperammonemia, elevated serum free fatty acids, and salicylate (aspirin) ingestion.

7-14. The answer is a. (*DiPalma, 4/e, pp 778–779. Hardman and Limbird, 9/e, pp 977–978.*) Primaquine is effective against the extraerythrocytic forms of *P. vivax* and *P. ovale* and is thus of value in a radical cure of malarial infection.

It also attacks the sexual forms of the parasite, rendering them incapable of maturation in the mosquito and making it valuable in preventing the spread of malarial infection.

7-15. The answer is d. *(Burkitt, 3/e, p 352. Junqueira, 8/e, pp 440–442. Yen, 3/e, pp 837–839.)* The patient described in this question is probably pregnant. The delay in menstruation coupled with the presence of basophilic cells in a vaginal smear is a clue. Ovulation is the midpoint of the cycle and should be more than a few days away. She is relatively young for the onset of menopause and there are no other symptoms. The vaginal epithelium varies little with the normal menstrual cycle. Exfoliative cytology can be used to diagnose cancer and to determine if the epithelium is under stimulation of estrogen and progesterone. The presence of basophilic cells in the smear with the Pap staining method would indicate the presence of both estrogen and progesterone. The data suggest the maintenance of the corpus luteum (i.e., pregnancy).

7-16. The answer is b. *(Cotran, 5/e, pp 601–603.)* Paroxysmal nocturnal hemoglobinuria (PNH) is an acquired clonal stem cell disorder that is characterized by abnormal red cells, granulocytes, and platelets. The red blood cells (RBCs) are abnormally sensitive to the lytic activity of complement due to a deficiency of GPI (glycosyl phosphatidyl inositol) linked proteins, namely decay-accelerating factor (DAF, or CD55), membrane inhibitor of reactive lysis (CD55), or CD59 (a C8 binding protein). Complement is normally activated by acidotic states, such as occurs with exercise or sleep. In patients with PNH, the acidotic condition that develops during sleep (which is usually at night) causes hemolysis of red blood cells and results in a red urine in the morning. The erythrocytes of these patients lyse in vitro with acid (Ham's test) or sucrose (sucrose lysis test). Complications of PNH include the development of frequent thromboses, particularly of the hepatic, portal, or cerebral veins. Since PNH is a clonal stem cell disorder, patients are at an increased risk of developing aplastic anemia or acute leukemia.

Antibody-mediated destruction of red cells may be due to autoimmune reactions or isoimmune reactions. The latter is due to antibodies from one person which react with RBCs from another person. This isoimmune destruction is seen with blood transfusions and hemolytic disease of the newborn. The autoimmune hemolytic anemias (AIHA) are hemolytic anemias that are due to the presence of antibodies that destroy red cells. The AIHAs are divided into two main types: those secondary to "warm" antibodies and those reactive at cold temperatures. Warm-antibody autoimmune hemolytic anemias react at 37° C in vitro, are composed of IgG, and do not fix complement. Instead, immunoglobulin-coated RBCs are removed by splenic macrophages that recognize the Fc portion of the immunoglobulin. These warm IgG antibodies are found in patients with malignant tumors, especially leukemia-lymphoma; they are associated with the use of such drugs as a methyldopa; and are also found in the autoimmune diseases, especially lupus erythematosus. Cold-antibody autoimmune hemolytic anemia (cold AIHA) is subdivided into two clinical categories based on the type of antibody that is involved. These two types of cold antibodies are cold agglutinins and cold hemolysins. Cold agglutinins are monoclonal IgM antibodies that react at 4 to 6° C. They are called agglutinins because the IgM can agglutinate red cells due to its large size (pentamer). Additionally, IgM can activate complement, which may result in IV hemolysis. Two diseases are classically associated with cold agglutinin formation. They are mycoplasma pneumonitis and infectious mononucleosis. In contrast, cold hemolysins are seen in patients with PCH (paroxysmal cold hemoglobinuria). These cold hemolysins are unique because they are biphasic anti-erythrocyte autoantibodies. These antibodies are IgG that is directed against the "P" blood group antigen. They are called biphasic because they attach to red cells and bind complement at low temperatures, but the activation of complement does not occur until the temperature is increased. This antibody, called the Donath-Landsteiner antibody, was previously associated with syphilis, but may follow various infections, such as mycoplasmal pneumonia.

7-17. The answer is b. (*Cotran, 5/e, pp 217–218, 1166.*) The branchial apparatus consists of the branchial clefts (ectoderm), the branchial arches (mesoderm and neural crest), and the branchial (pharyngeal) pouches (endoderm). The third pouch (dorsal wings) develops into the inferior parathyroid glands; the third pouch (ventral wings) develop into the thymus; the fourth pouch develops into the superior parathyroids; while the fifth pouch develops into the ultimobranchial bodies, which in turn gives rise to the C cells of the thyroid. DiGeorge's syndrome results from a failure of the development of the third and fourth pharyngeal pouches. This abnormality is associated with tetany and an absence of T cells. The tetany results from the hypocalcemia caused by the lack of the parathyroid glands, while the absence of T cells is caused by the lack of the thymus gland.

7-18. The answer is e. *(McPhee, 2/e, pp 531–535; Fauci, 14/e, pp 2105–2107.)* Hypothyroid patients tend to gain weight. Prolactin-secreting tumors (prolactinomas), being located in the pituitary, would be expected to show abnormal physical exam findings at the eyes, given that the tumor typically sits on the optic chiasma. Early menopause is unlikely in a 22-year-old. Resistance to LH and FSH would have prohibited this patient from ever having menses. This leaves excessive exercise as the only remaining plausible cause in this patient.

7-19. The answer is d. *(Cotran, 5/e, p 397. Rubin, 2/e, pp 308–313.)* Many environmental chemicals are potential causes of quite serious human diseases. Cyanide causes cellular damage by binding to cytochrome oxidase and inhibiting cellular respiration. It is a component of amygdalin, which is found in the pits of several fruits, such as apricots and peaches. Cyanide poisoning is betrayed by the presence of the odor of bitter almonds. Ethylene glycol, commonly used as an antifreeze, is toxic to humans. It causes acute tubular necrosis in the kidney. Carbon monoxide replaces oxygen in hemoglobin and causes the formation of carboxyhemoglobin and anoxia. Despite the extreme cyanosis, it produces a characteristic cherry-red color to the skin. Mercury toxicity damages both the kidney (proximal tubular necrosis) and the brain. The neurologic symptoms include mental changes and a tremor. Mercury was used in the hat industry, and the symptoms of toxicity resulted in the expression "mad as a hatter." Methanol, originally called "wood alcohol," is metabolized in the body to formaldehyde and formic acid. These metabolites cause necrosis of retinal ganglion cells, which produces blindness.

7-20. The answer is a. *(Cotran, 5/e, pp 956–957, 960.)* Many diseases involve hematuria, and a few diseases occur in the setting of an upper respiratory infection or of upper respiratory signs and symptoms. When the hematuria follows within 2 days of the onset of an upper respiratory infection without skin lesions in a young patient, IgA nephropathy (Berger's disease) should be considered. This disease involves the deposition of IgA in the mesangium of the glomeruli. Light microscopic examination may suggest the disease, but renal biopsy immunofluorescence (IF) must be performed to confirm it. This disorder may be the most common cause of the nephritic syndrome worldwide. The hematuria may become recurrent, with proteinuria that may approach nephrotic syndrome proportions. Serum levels of IgA may be elevated. A small percentage of patients may progress to renal failure over a period of years. In contrast to Berger's disease, a linear IF pattern suggests a type II hypersensitivity reaction, such as Goodpasture's disease, while a granular pattern is seen with post-streptococcal glomerulonephritis (GN), membranous GN, focal segmental glomerulosclerosis, and membranoproliferative GN. Most positive immunofluorescence patterns involve IgG and C3, except that a granular IgM pattern is present in focal segmental glomerulosclerosis, while mesangial IgA is seen in IgA nephropathy (Berger's disease). Lipoid nephrosis would have a negative IF pattern; that is, there would be no staining present.

7-21. The answer is e. (*Cotran, 5/e, pp 649–654.*) The leukemias are malignant neoplasms of the hematopoietic stem cells that are characterized by diffuse replacement of the bone marrow by neoplastic cells. These malignant cells frequently spill into the peripheral blood. The leukemias are divided into acute and chronic forms, and then further subdivided based on lymphocytic or myelocytic (myelogenous) forms. Thus, the four basic patterns of acute leukemia are: acute lymphocytic leukemia (ALL), chronic lymphocytic leukemia (CLL), acute myelocytic leukemia (AML), and chronic myelocytic leukemia (CML).

Acute leukemias are characterized by a decrease in the mature forms of cells and an increase in the immature forms (leukemic blasts). Acute leukemias, both ALL and AML, have an abrupt clinical onset and present with symptoms due to failure of normal marrow function. Symptoms include fever (secondary to an infection), easy fatigability (due to anemia), and bleeding (due to thrombocytopenia). The peripheral smear in patients with acute leukemia reveals the white cell count to usually be increased. The peripheral smear also reveals signs of anemia and thrombocytopenia. More importantly, however, there are blasts in the peripheral smear. The diagnosis of acute leukemia is made by finding more than 30 percent blasts in the bone marrow.

AML primarily affects adults between the ages of 15 and 39 and is characterized by the neoplastic proliferation of myeloblasts. Myeloblasts, characterized by their delicate nuclear chromatin, may contain 3 to 5 nucleoli. Myeloblasts in some cases of AML have distinct intracytoplasmic rod-like structures that stain red and are called Auer rods. These are abnormal lysosomal structures (primary granules) that are considered pathognomonic of myeloblasts. AML is divided into seven types by the French-American-British (FAB) classification:

M1—myeloblastic leukemia without maturation (cells are mainly blasts)

M2—myeloblastic leukemia with maturation (some promyelocytes are present)

M3—hypergranular promyelocytic leukemia (numerous granules and many Auer rods)

M4—myelomonocytic leukemia (both myeloblasts and monoblasts)

M5—monocytic leukemia (infiltrates in the gingiva are characteristic)

M6—erythroleukemia (Di Guglielmo's disease)

M7—acute megakaryocytic leukemia (associated with myelofibrosis)

Acute promyelocytic leukemia (M3 AML) is characterized by several specific features that are found in no other types of acute leukemia. There are numerous abnormal promyelocytes present that have numerous cytoplasmic granules and numerous Auer rods. If these numerous granules are released from dying cells, which may occur with treatment, they may activate extensive, uncontrolled intravascular coagulation and cause the development of DIC (disseminated intravascular coagulation). This abnormality is characterized by increased fibrin degradation products in the blood. M3 AML is also characterized by the translocation t(15;17), which results in the fusion of the retinoic acid receptor-alpha gene on chromosome 17 to the PML unit on chromosome 15. This produces an abnormal retinoic acid receptor and provides the basis for treatment of these patients with all-trans-retinoic acid.

7-22. The answer is a. (*Cotran, 5/e, pp 499–504.*) An aneurysm is an abnormal dilatation of any vessel. The causes of aneurysms are many, but the two most important are atherosclerosis and cystic medial necrosis. Atherosclerotic aneurysms, the most common type of aortic aneurysm, usually occur distal to the renal arteries and proximal to the bifurcation of the aorta.

Many atherosclerotic aneurysms are asymptomatic, but if they rupture they will produce sudden, severe abdominal pain, shock, and a risk of death. Prior to rupture, physical examination reveals a pulsatile mass in the abdomen. Cystic medial necrosis refers to the focal loss of elastic and muscle fibers in the media of vessels and is seen in patients with hypertension, dissecting aneurysms, and Marfan's syndrome. Trauma may also lead to the formation of dissecting aneurysms.

Berry aneurysms, found at the bifurcation of arteries in the circle of Willis, are due to congenital defects in the vascular wall. Syphilitic (luetic) aneurysms are caused by obliterative endarteritis of the vasa vasorum of the aorta. These luetic aneurysms are part of the tertiary manifestation of syphilis and become evident 15 to 20 years after persons have contracted the initial infection with *Treponema pallidum*. Elastic tissue and smooth muscle cells of the media undergo ischemic destruction as a result of the treponemal infection (obliterative endarteritis). As a consequence of ischemia in the media, musculoelastic support is lost and fibrosis occurs. Grossly the aorta has a "tree-bark" appearance. Luetic aneurysm almost always occurs in the thoracic aorta and may lead to luetic heart disease by producing insufficiency of the aortic valve (aortic regurgitation).

7-23. The answer is c. (*Wilson-Pauwels, p 88. Adam, pp 1376–1377.*) This is an example of Bell's palsy, or damage to the facial nerve distal to its nucleus in the pons. The motor weakness is lower motor neuron because of the involvement of the upper one-third of the face (this has bilateral innervation within the central nervous system). The loss of taste on the anterior two-thirds of the tongue and the hyperacusis (sensitivity to noise) point to damage distal to the brainstem because these are functions whose nerves join the facial nerve distal to its exit from the pons. This type of palsy may be caused by a virus and is more common among people with diabetes.

7-24. The answer is e. (*Wilson-Pauwels, p 88.*) This type of facial paralysis, involving the upper one-third of the facial muscles, is characteristic of a lower motor neuron facial nerve lesion. Since there is bilateral innervation within the central nervous system, from the prefrontal gyrus bilaterally, until their synapse at the facial nerve nucleus, all upper motor neuron facial weakness spares the forehead.

7-25. The answer is e. (*Wilson-Pauwels, p 94. Kandel, 3/e, p 691.*) Since there is motor weakness of the face, and the chorda tympani nerve, which subserves taste, joins the facial nerve, it is likely that the lesion exists proximal to where the chorda tympani joins the facial nerve. A lesion in the lingual nerve (a branch of the trigeminal) would result in a loss of taste, as well, but would also result in a loss of sensation to the face, not motor weakness. If the lesion occurred distal to the chorda tympani nerve, taste would have been spared.

7-26. The answer is e. (*Wilson-Pauwels, p 86. Kandel, 3/e, p 691. Adams, p 1376. Noback, p 236.*) The facial nerve sends a branch to the stapedius muscle distal to the geniculate ganglion, but proximal to the chorda tympani nerve. Lesions proximal to this branch will cause weakness of the stapedius muscle. Contraction of this muscle normally serves as a mechanism for dampening the motion of the ossicles, thus lowering the amount of stimulation reaching the Organ of Corti. If this muscle is paralyzed, hyperacusis (increased acuity) as well as hypersensitivity to low tones will occur.

7-27. The answer is d. (*Sierles, pp 181–184.*) In an initial interview with a patient it is important to give a high priority to establishing a good doctor-patient relationship in order to facilitate good communication. With this patient it is important to introduce yourself, as this can have a calming effect on an emotionally upset patient if it is done in a reassuring and confident tone of voice. Since this patient is upset and has already told you that his father died with similar symptoms only two years ago, it is probably best to calmly inquire about family history of heart disease. Usually, such a patient will begin to calm down, will address your question, and you will have begun to establish a good cooperative doctor-patient relationship with positive communication. Immediately attempting to reassure the patient that his pain is not related to his father's illness is apt to be aggravating, since he will surmise that you don't really know that. Inquiring about his father's pain is not immediately helpful in reaching your diagnosis, and ordering an emergency electrocardiogram is premature at this point. Asking a number of direct medical questions is also premature for an excited patient until after you have established a more stable communication.

7-28. The answer is b. (*Levinson, Jawetz, 4/e, pp 130–132.*) This patient appears to have primary syphilis as evidenced by a penile chancre that was not tender. One of the differences between syphilis and herpes simplex virus (HSV) is that an HSV lesion is excruciatingly painful. Treponemal organisms may be seen microscopically in the lesion if the lesion is scraped. If not treated, the chancre will disappear and the patient will be asymptomatic until he/she exhibits the signs/symptoms of secondary syphilis, which include a disseminated rash and systemic involvement such as meningitis, hepatitis, or nephritis. There are two kinds of tests for the detection of syphilis antibodies: nonspecific tests such as the RPR and VDRL, and specific tests such as the FTA, TPHA (*Treponema pallidum* hemagglutination test), and the MHTP (microhemagglutination *T. pallidum*). The difference is that the nonspecific tests use a cross-reactive antigen known as cardiolipin, while the specific tests use a *T. pallidum* antigen. Although the nonspecific tests are sensitive, they lack specificity and often cross-react in patients who have diabetes, hepatitis, infectious mononucleosis, or who are pregnant. Some patients, especially those with autoimmune diseases, will have both nonspecific (RPR) and specific tests (FTA) positive. Resolution of such a situation can be done by molecular methods for *T. pallidum* such as PCR, or by the immobilization test using live spirochetes and the patient's serum. In the TPI test the spirochetes will die in the presence of specific antibody.

7-29. The answer is c. (*Fauci, 14/e, p 627.*) The definitive diagnosis is superior vena cava syndrome until proven otherwise with scans.

7-30. The answer is a. (*Cotran, 5/e, pp 562–566. Rubin, 2/e, pp 543–545.*) Inflammation of the myocardium, myocarditis, has numerous causes, but most of the well-documented cases of myocarditis are of viral origin. The most common viral causes are coxsackieviruses A and B, ECHO virus, and influenza virus. Patients usually develop symptoms a few weeks after a viral infection. Most patients recover from the acute myocarditis, but a few may die from congestive heart failure or arrhythmias. Sections of the heart will show patchy or diffuse interstitial infiltrates composed of T lymphocytes and macrophages. There may be focal or patchy acute myocardial necrosis. Bacterial infections of the myocardium produce multiple foci of inflammation composed mainly of neutrophils. Giant cell myocarditis, which was previously called Fiedler's myocarditis, is characterized by granulomatous inflammation with giant cells and is usually rapidly fatal. In hypersensitivity myocarditis, which is caused by hypersensitivity reactions to several drugs, the inflammatory infiltrate includes many eosinophils, and the infiltrate is both interstitial and perivascular. Beriberi, one of the metabolic diseases of the heart, is a cause of high-output failure and is characterized by decreased peripheral vascular resistance and increased cardiac output. Patients have dilated hearts, but the microscopic changes are nonspecific. Hyperthyroid disease and Paget's disease are other causes of high-output failure.

7-31. The answer is b. *(Cotran, 5/e, pp 340–341, 349–350. Chandrasoma, 3/e, p 805.)* The cytopathic effect of viruses is often a clue to the diagnosis of the type of infection that is present. There are several types of herpes viruses, which are relatively large, double-stranded DNA viruses. Infection by herpes simplex virus (HSV) or varicella-zoster virus (VZV) is recognized by nuclear homogenization (ground-glass nuclei), intranuclear inclusions (Cowdry type A bodies), and the formation of multinucleated cells. Herpes simplex type 2, a sexually transmitted viral disease, results in the formation of vesicles that ulcerate and cause burning, itching, and pain. These lesions will heal spontaneously, but the virus will remain dormant in the lumbar and sacral ganglia. Recurrent infections may occur, and transmission to the newborn during delivery is a feared complication that may be fatal to the infant. Shingles and chickenpox are caused by herpes zoster, which is identical to varicella.

Cytomegalovirus (CMV) causes both the nucleus and the cytoplasm of infected cells to be enlarged. Infected cells have large, purple intranuclear inclusions surrounded by a clear halo and smaller, less prominent basophilic intracytoplasmic inclusions. Adenoviruses can produce similar inclusions, but the infected cells are not enlarged. They also produce characteristic smudge cells in infected respiratory epithelial cells. Human papilloma virus (HPV) infection may produce a characteristic effect that is called koilocytosis. Histologic examination reveals enlarged squamous epithelial cells that have shrunken nuclei ("raisin-oid") within large cytoplasmic vacuoles.

Candidiasis is the most common fungal infection of the vagina, especially common in patients with diabetes or taking oral contraceptives. Candida infection causes vulvar itching and produces a white discharge. Microscopic examination of the vaginal discharge reveals yeast and pseudohyphae. *Trichomonas vaginalis*, a large, pear-shaped, flagellated protozoan, causes severe vaginal itching with dysuria. It produces a thick yellow-gray discharge.

7-32. The answer is c. *(Katzung, 7/e, pp 203–204.)* Overloading of cell Ca leads to "delayed afterdepolarizations." These afterpotentials can interfere with normal conduction by further reducing the resting potential; if they regularly reach threshold in the conduction system, an arrhythmia can occur.

7-33. The answer is a. *(Fauci, 14/e, p 1975.)* Medications are important in the differential diagnosis of hyperprolactinemia. A common drug that causes increased prolactin with possible amenorrhea and galactorrhea is haloperidol, a dopamine antagonist. Lisinopril has no effect on prolactin levels. The antidepressants fluoxetin and amitriptyline and anxiolytic buspirone may cause small changes in prolactin levels but rarely enough to cause a clinical syndrome.

7-34. The answer is d. *(McPhee, 2/e, pp 527–528; Fauci, 14/e, p 2012.)* In both premenopausal and menopausal women, androgen levels may be normal or high, estrogen levels normal, and the prolactin level normal. Androgen production can be in the ovary or the adrenal gland. Estrogen production is mainly in the ovary prior to menopause and in the periphery by conversion of testosterone in menopause. The amount of estrogen during menopause is a function of the patient's amount of adipose tissue. High FSH and LH levels are the hallmarks of a lack of adequate ovarian production of both estrogen and progesterone, the chemical markers of menopause, due to lack of negative feedback.

7-35. The answer is c. *(April, 3/e, pp 383–384.)* The umbilical region is innervated by the tenth intercostal nerve. The afferent nerve fibers from the jejunum and ileum as well as from the ascending colon and transverse colon travel through the superior mesenteric plexus and along the lesser splanchnic nerve to spinal nerves T10 and T11. Thus, pain originating from these portions of the gastrointestinal tract will refer pain to the umbilical region. The ascending colon and descending colon, which are secondarily retroperitoneal, are unlikely to be involved in the umbilical herniation. The mobile transverse colon could be involved, but the referred pain would tend to be subumbilical, not periumbilical.

7-36. The answer is c. *(Levinson, Jawetz, 4/e, p 283.)* *Acanthamoeba* is a free living amoeba as is *Naegleria*. *Naegleria* usually causes severe, often fatal meningoencephalitis, while *Acanthamoeba* is uncommonly isolated from contact lens fluid and patients with retinitis who do not store their lenses under sterile conditions. *Acanthamoeba* can be grown on nonnutrient agar plates using *E. coli* as a food source. They are identified microscopically by use of a nonspecific fluorescent stain.

7-37. The answer is a. *(Damjanov, 10/e, pp 2273–2275. Rubin, 2/e, p 946.)* "Fibroids" of the uterus are among the most common abnormalities seen in uteri surgically removed in the United States in women of reproductive age. They arise in the myometrium, submucosally, subserosally, and midwall, both singly and several at a time. Sharply circumscribed, they are benign, smooth muscle tumors that are firm, gray-white, and whorled on cut section. Their malignant counterpart, leiomyosarcoma of the uterus, is quite rare in the de novo state and arises even more rarely from an antecedent leiomyoma. Whereas cell pleomorphism, tissue necrosis, and cytologic atypia per se are established criteria in assessing malignancy in tumors generally, they are important to the pathologist in uterine fibroids only if mitoses are also present. Regardless of cellularity or atypicality, if 10 or more mitoses are present in 10 separate high-power microscopic fields, the lesion is leiomyosarcoma. If 5 or fewer mitoses are present in 10 fields with bland morphology, the leiomyoma will behave in a benign fashion. Problems arise when the mitotic counts range between 3 and 7 per 10 fields with varying degrees of cell and tissue atypicality. These equivocal lesions should be regarded by both pathologist and clinician as "gray-area" smooth muscle tumors of unpredictable biologic behavior. Fortunately, the "gray-area" leiomyoma of the uterus is rarely seen. Thus mitoses are the most important criteria in assessing malignancy in smooth muscle tumors of the uterus.

7-38 The answer is d. *(Adams, 6/e, p 280, 538.)* Herb's drooping eyelid, small pupil, and lack of sweating on the right side are examples of Horner syndrome. This is caused by the interruption of sympathetic fibers anywhere along their course from the hypothalamus and brainstem to the intermediolateral cell column in the upper thoracic levels of the spinal cord where neurons, supplying sympathetic innervation to the pupil, the levator palpebrae superioris muscle of the eyelid, and sweat glands of the face, are located.

7-39. The answer is a. *(Adams, 6/e, p 280, 538.)* Interruption of this sympathetic innervation will result in the drooping of the upper eyelid (ptosis), pupillary constriction (miosis; due to unopposed action of the parasympathetic innervation of the circular muscles of the iris), and lack of sweating on the face. Parasympathetic or oculomotor damage causes pupillary dilation, rather than constriction.

7-40. The answer is c. *(Kandel, 3/e, p 692.)* Herb could close his eyes tightly because this function is mediated by the seventh nerve, which is not damaged by this lesion.

7-41. The answer is e. *(Kandel, 3/e, pp 762–770. Adams, 6/e, p 280.)* Preganglionic sympathetic neurons are predominantly cholinergic and postganglionic sympathetic neurons are predominantly noradrenergic. Horner syndrome may be caused by either a preganglionic or postganglionic lesion. The location may be determined by the use of eyedrops specifically targeted at a particular neurotransmitter.

7-42. The answer is a. *(Cotran, 5/e, pp 326–327. Damjanov, 10/e, pp 850–854.)* There are several types of mycobacteria that are not M. *tuberculosis.* These organisms are called atypical mycobacteria, or mycobacteria other than tuberculosis (MOTT). They are separated into different classes (Runyon classes) based on several culture characteristics, such as pigment production, colony morphology, and rate of growth. Examples of MOTT include M. *avium-intracellulare,* M. *marinum,* and M. *leprae,* which is the causative agent of leprosy. M. *avium-intracellulare* is an important cause of infection in patients with AIDS. Histologic sections in these immunosuppressed patients do not reveal granulomas because the cellular immune reactions of these patients are defective. Instead numerous organisms can be seen with special stains. M. *marinum* inhabits marine organisms and grows in water. It can cause superficial disease, skin and subcutaneous disease and can be obtained from infected aquariums or swimming pools.

7-43. The answer is a. *(Katzung, 7/e, p 493.)* Of the listed antidepressants, only amitriptyline, a tricyclic, causes adverse effects related to blockade of muscarinic acetylcholine receptors. Both trazodone and amitriptyline cause adverse effects related to α-adrenoreceptor blockade.

7-44. The answer is a. *(Cotran, 5/e, pp 683–692.)* Chronic obstructive pulmonary diseases (COPD) are characterized by obstruction to airflow somewhere along the airways. These diseases may affect the bronchus, the bronchiole, or the acinus. Asthma, bronchiectasis, and chronic bronchitis affect primarily the bronchus, while emphysema affects primarily the acinus. Asthma is a pulmonary disease that is caused by excessive bronchoconstriction secondary to airways that are hyper-reactive to numerous stimuli. Asthma has been divided into extrinsic and intrinsic categories. The extrinsic category includes atopic (allergic) asthma, occupational asthma, and allergic bronchopulmonary aspergillosis. The intrinsic category includes non-reaginic asthma and pharmacologic asthma. The former is related to respiratory tract infections, while the latter is often related to aspirin sensitivity. These aspirin-sensitive patients often have recurrent rhinitis and nasal polyps. In these patients the aspirin initiates an asthmatic attack by inhibiting the cyclooxygenase pathway of arachidonic acid metabolism without affecting the lipoxygenase pathway. This causes the relative excess production of the leukotrienes, which are bronchoconstrictors.

7-45. The answer is b. *(Cotran, 5/e, pp 746–747. Rubin, 2/e, pp 1266–1271.)* Ménière's disease is an abnormality that is characterized by periodic episodes of vertigo, which are often accompanied by nausea and vomiting, sensorineural hearing loss, and tinnitus (ringing in the ears). These symptoms are related to hydropic dilatation of the endolymphatic system of the cochlea. Inflammation of the middle ear (otitis media), which occurs most often in children, may be acute or chronic. If caused by viruses, there may be a serous exudate, but if produced by bacteria, there may be a suppurative exudate. Acute suppurative otitis media is characterized by acute suppurative inflammation (neutrophils), while chronic otitis media has chronic inflammation with granulation tissue. Chronic otitis media may cause perforation of the eardrum or may lead to the formation of a cyst within the middle ear that is filled with keratin. This cyst is called a cholesteatoma. The name is somewhat of a misnomer as cholesterol deposits are not present. Otosclerosis, a common hereditary cause of bilateral conduction hearing loss, is associated with new spongy bone formation around the stapes and the oval window. Patients present with progressive deafness. Tumors of the middle ear are quite rare, but a neoplasm that arises from the paraganglia of the middle ear (the glomus jugulare or glomus tympanicum) is called a chemodectoma. Other names for this tumor include nonchromaffin paraganglioma and glomus jugulare tumor. This lesion is characterized histologically by lobules of cells in a highly vascular stroma (zellballen). A similar tumor that occurs in the neck is called a carotid body tumor.

7-46. The answer is b. *(Fauci, 14/e, p 1985.)* This patient presents with clinical manifestations of hypothyroidism, with a low free T$_4$. Secondary hypothyroidism is suggested by the low TSH. The diagnostic test of choice is an MRI of the pituitary for evaluation of a possible pituitary tumor.

7-47. The answer is c. *(Mandell, 3/e, p 1547.)* Bruton's agammaglobulinemia is a congenital defect that becomes apparent at approximately 6 months of age when maternal IgG is diminished. The child is unable to produce immunoglobulins and develops a series of bacterial infections characterized by recurrences and progression to more serious infections such as septicemia. Cell-mediated immunity is not affected and the child is able to respond normally to diseases that require this immune response for resolution.

7-48. The answer is b. *(Cotran, 5/e, pp 1081–1086.)* Gestational trophoblastic diseases include the benign hydatidiform mole (partial and complete), the invasive mole (chorioadenoma destruens), placental site trophoblastic tumor, and choriocarcinoma. Hydatidiform moles are composed of avascular, grape-like structures that do not invade the myometrium. In complete (classic) moles, all the chorionic villi are abnormal and fetal parts are not found. They have a 46,XX diploid pattern and arise from the paternal chromosomes of a single sperm by a process called androgenesis. In partial moles, only some of the villi are abnormal and fetal parts may be seen. These moles have a triploid or a tetraploid karyotype and arise from the fertilization of a single egg by two sperm. About 2 percent of complete moles may develop into chorio-carcinoma, but partial moles are rarely followed by malignancy. The invasive mole penetrates the myometrium and may even embolize to distant sites. A similar lesion is the placental site trophoblastic tumor, which is characterized by invasion of the myometrium by intermediate trophoblasts. Gestational choriocarcinomas, composed of malignant proliferations of both cytotro-phoblasts and syncytiotrophoblasts without the formation of villi, can arise from either normal or abnormal pregnancies; 50 percent arise in hydatidiform moles, 25 percent in previous abortions, 22 percent in normal pregnancies, and the rest in ectopic pregnancies or teratomas. Both hydatidiform moles and choriocarcinomas have high levels of human chorionic gonadotropin (hCG);

the levels are extremely high in choriocarcinoma unless considerable tumor necrosis is present.

7-49. The answer is e. (*Cotran, 5/e, pp 264–265.*) There are several mechanisms by which proto-oncogenes (p-oncs) can become oncogenic (c-oncs). Normal cellular genes (proto-oncogenes) may become oncogenic by being incorporated into the viral genome (forming v-oncs), or they may be activated by other processes to form cellular oncogenes (c-oncs). These other processes include gene mutations, chromosomal translocations, and gene amplifications. Gene mutations, such as point mutations, are associated with the formation of cancers by mutant *c-ras* oncogenes. This abnormality is found in many visceral adenocarcinomas.

Chromosomal translocations are associated with the development of many types of cancers, one example of which is Burkitt's lymphoma. The most common translocation associated with Burkitt's lymphoma is t(8;14), in which the *c-myc* oncogene on chromosome 8 is brought in contact with the immunoglobulin heavy chain gene on chromosome 14. Two other examples of chromosomal translocations are the association of chronic myelocytic leukemia (CML) with t(9;22), which is the Philadelphia chromosome, and the association of follicular lymphoma with the translocation t(18;14). The former involves the proto-oncogene *c-abl*, which is rearranged in proximity to a break point cluster region (bcr) on chromosome 22. The resultant chimeric *c-abl/bcr* gene encodes a protein with tyrosine kinase activity. The t(18;14) involves the *bcl-2* oncogene on chromosome 18. Expression of the oncogene *bcl-2* is associated with the prevention of apoptosis in germinal centers. Examples of associations that involve gene amplification include *N-myc* and neuroblastoma, *c-neu* and breast cancer, and *erb-B* and breast and ovarian cancers. Gene amplification can be demonstrated by finding doublet minutes or homogenous staining regions.

7-50. The answer is e. (*Murray, 24/e.*) The major problem in myasthenia gravis is a marked reduction of acetylcholine receptors on the motor endplate where cranial nerves form a neuromuscular junction with muscles. In these patients, autoantibodies against the acetylcholine receptors effectively reduce their numbers. Normally, acetylcholine molecules released by the nerve terminal bind to receptors on the muscle endplate, resulting in a stimulation of contraction by depolarizing the muscle membrane. The condition is improved with drugs that inhibit acetylcholinesterase.

BIBLIOGRAPHY

Abenhaim L, Moride Y, Brenot F, et al: Appetite-suppressant drugs and the risk of primary pulmonary hypertension. *N Engl J Med* 335(9): 609–16, 1996.

Adams RD, Victor M, Ropper, AH: *Principles of Neurology*, 6/e. New York, McGraw-Hill, 1997.

Alberts B, Bray D, Lewis J, et al: *Molecular Biology of the Cell*, 3/e. New York, Garland, 1994.

April EW: *Clinical Anatomy*, 3/e. New York, John Wiley & Sons, 1997.

Baron S: *Medical Microbiology*, 4/e. New York, Churchill Livingstone, 1996.

Barron WM, Lindheimer MD: *Medical Disorders During Pregnancy*, 2d ed. St. Louis, CV Mosby, 1995.

Baum A, Gatchel RJ, Krantz DS: *An Introduction to Health Psychology*, 3/e. New York, McGraw-Hill, 1997.

Burkitt HG, Young B, Heath JW: *Wheater's Functional Histology*, 3/e. New York, Churchill Livingstone, 1993.

Chandrasoma P, Taylor CR: *Concise Pathology*, 3/e. East Norwalk, CT, Appleton & Lange, 1998.

Coe FL, Favus MJ (eds): *Disorders of Bone and Mineral Metabolism*. New York, Raven, 1992.

Connolly HM, Crary JL, et al: Valvular heart disease associated with fenfluramine-phentermine. *N Engl J Med* 337(9): 581–8, 1997.

Cotran RS, Kumar V, Robbins SL: *Robbins' Pathologic Basis of Disease*, 5/e. Philadelphia, Saunders, 1994.

Damjanov I, Linder J (eds): *Anderson's Pathology*, 10/e. St. Louis, Mosby, 1996.

Davis BD, et al: *Microbiology*, 4/e. New York, Harper & Row, 1990.

DiPalma JR, DiGregorio GJ, Barbieri EJ, Ferko AP: *Basic Pharmacology in Medicine*, 4/e. West Chester, PA, Medical Surveillance, 1994.

Duchin JS, et al: Hantavirus pulmonary syndrome: A clinical description of 17 patients with a newly recognized disease. *N Engl J Med* 330:949–955, 1994.

Fauci AS, Braunwald E, Isselbacher KJ, Wilson JD, Martin JB, Kasper DL, Hauser SL, Longo DL (eds): *Harrison's Principles of Internal Medicine*, 14th ed. New York, McGraw-Hill, 1998.

Gelehrter TD, Collins FS: *Principles of Medical Genetics*. Baltimore, Williams & Wilkins, 1990.

Greenspan FS: *Basic and Clinical Endocrinology*, 5/e. East Norwalk, CT, Appleton & Lange, 1997.

Hardman JG, Limbird LE (eds): *Goodman & Gilman's the Pharmacological Basis of Therapeutics*, 9/e. New York, McGraw-Hill, 1996.

Henry JB, et al (eds): *Clinical Diagnosis and Management by Laboratory Methods*, 19/e. Philadelphia, Saunders, 1996.

Howard BJ, Keiser JF, Smith TF, Weissfeld AS, Tilton RC: *Clinical and Pathogenic Microbiology*, 2/e. St. Louis, Mosby, 1993.

Isselbacher KJ, Braunwald E, Wilson JD, Martin JB, Fauci AS, Kasper DL (eds): *Harrison's Principles of Internal Medicine*, 13/e. New York, McGraw-Hill, 1994.

Jawetz E, Melnick JL, Adelbert EA: *Review of Medical Microbiology*, 19/e. East Norwalk, CT, Appleton & Lange, 1991.

Joklik WK et al (eds): *Zinsser Microbiology*, 20/e. East Norwalk, CT, Appleton & Lange, 1992.

Jorde LB, Carey JC, White RL: *Medical Genetics*. St. Louis, Mosby, 1995.

Junqueira LC, Carneiro J, Kelley RO: *Basic Histology,* 8/e. East Norwalk, CT, Appleton & Lange, 1995.

Kandel ER, Schwartz JH, Jessel TM: *Principles of Neural Science,* 3/e. New York, Elsevier, 1991.

Katzung BG: *Basic and Clinical Pharmacology,* 7/e. East Norwalk, CT, Appleton & Lange, 1997.

Larsen WJ: *Human Embryology.* New York, Churchill Livingstone, 1993.

Levinson W, Jawetz E: *Medical Microbiology and Immunology,* 4/e. East Norwalk CT, Appleton & Lange, 1997.

Mandell GL, Douglas RG, Bennett JE: *Principles and Practice of Infectious Disease,* 3/e. New York, Wiley, 1990.

McPhee SJ, Lingappa VR, Ganong WF, Lange JD (eds): *Pathophysiology of Disease: An Introduction to Clinical Medicine,* 2d ed. East Norwarlk, CT, Appleton & Lange, 1997.

Moore KL: *The Developing Human: Clinically Oriented Embryology,* 5/e. Philadelphia, Saunders, 1993.

Murray PR, Rosenthal KS, Kobayashi GS, Pfaller MA: *Medical Microbiology,* 5th ed. St. Louis, CV Mosby, 1997.

Murray RK, Granner DK, Mayes PA, Rodwell, VW: Harper's *Biochemistry,* 24/e. East Norwalk, CT, Appleton & Lange, 1996.

Noback CR, Strominger NL, Demarest RJ: *The Human Nervous System,* 5/e. Baltimore, Williams & Wilkins, 1996.

Nolte J: *The Human Brain: An Introduction to its Functional Anatomy,* 4/e. St. Louis, Mosby, 1998.

Rhoades R. *Human Physiology,* 3/e. Orlando, Harcourt, 1995.

Ross MH, Romrell LJ, Kaye GI: *Histology: A Test Atlas,* 3/e. Baltimore, Williams & Wilkins, 1995.

Rowland LP (ed): *Merritt's Textbook of Neurology,* 9/e. Baltimore, Williams & Wilkins, 1995.

Rubin E, Farber JL: *Pathology,* 2/e. Philadelphia, Lippincott, 1994.

Sadler TW: *Langman's Medical Embryology,* 7/e. Baltimore, Williams & Wilkins, 1995.

Scriver CR, Beaudet AL, Sly WS, Valle D (eds): *The Metabolic and Molecular Bases of Inherited Disease,* 7/e. New York, McGraw-Hill, 1995.

Sherris JC: *Medical Microbiology: An Introduction to Infectious Diseases,* 2/e. East Norwalk, CT, Appleton & Lange, 1992.

Sierles FS (ed): *Behavioral Science for Medical Students,* Baltimore, Williams & Wilkins, 1993.

Stryer L: *Biochemistry,* 4/e. New York, Freeman, 1995.

Thompson MW, McInnes RR, Willard HF: *Genetics in Medicine,* 5/e. Philadelphia, WB Saunders, 1991.

Wilson-Pauwels L, Akesson EJ, Stewart PA: *Cranial Nerves: Gross Anatomy and Clinical Comments.* Toronto, Decker, 1988.

Yen SSC, Jaffe RB: *Reproductive Endocrinology,* 3/e. Philadelphia, Saunders, 1991.

ISBN 0-07-135133-7

9 780071 351331

90000

MCGRAW-HILL:
CLINICAL VIGNETTES